BASIC MATH FOR H PROFESSIONALS

PROFESSIONALS

BASIC MATH FOR HEALTH PROFESSIONALS

First Edition

Prepared by

Jaime Nguyen, MD, MPH, MS
President, 3MD Education and
Director of Healthcare
Penn Foster Education
Scranton, PA

Elsevier
3251 Riverport Lane
St. Louis, Missouri 63043

Basic Math for Health Professionals, First Edition

ISBN: 978-0-323-76407-0

Notice

Practitioners and researchers must always rely on their own experience and knowledge in evaluating and using any information, methods, compounds or experiments described herein. Because of rapid advances in the medical sciences, in particular, independent verification of diagnoses and drug dosages should be made. To the fullest extent of the law, no responsibility is assumed by Elsevier, authors, editors or contributors for any injury and/or damage to persons or property as a matter of products liability, negligence or otherwise, or from any use or operation of any methods, products, instructions, or ideas contained in the material herein.

Senior Content Strategist: Luke Held
Director, Content Development: Laurie Gower
Content Development Specialist: John Tomedi
Publishing Services Manager: Deepthi Unni
Project Manager: Aparna Venkatachalam

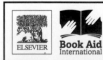

Printed in Canada

Last digit is the print number: 9 8 7 6 5 4 3 2 1

Preface

Welcome to *Basic Math for Health Professionals*. Regardless of one's role in the healthcare industry, all healthcare professionals will be required to demonstrate math competency in their job duties. This online course + workbook combination product is designed to help students establish a solid foundation of math skills and knowledge, giving them the confidence to perform more advanced calculations, both in school and in the workplace.

The online course introduces foundational math skills, such as types of numbers, as well as basic calculations: adding, subtracting, multiplying, and dividing whole numbers. From there, students progress to working with fractions, decimals, proportions, and percentages. They learn units of time and measurement, including the metric system, and practice converting between different units and measurement systems. Students can then use their new knowledge and skills reading drug labels, calculating parenteral dosages, and basic dosage by weight. Additionally, students will be able to conduct basic statistical analyses used in healthcare.

We have endeavored to create a product that provides a simple process for learning these math skills. Our goal is to make math as unintimidating and student-friendly as possible. The online course presents mathematical concepts using approachable explanations. Students can view narrated videos showing step-by-step solutions to calculations, and complete math activities with instant feedback.

After presenting the material and giving an opportunity to practice, the course directs the student to specific exercises in this worktext. Students first tackle the Practice Exercises using their newfound skills, and the book directs students to the specific screen of the online course containing detailed, step-by-step solutions to the problems. Practice Drills follow these exercises in the worktext, providing hundreds of problems to calculate "by hand." Finally, the worktext chapters end with a set of comprehensive Review Questions. Answers to all the Practice Drills and Review Questions are found in the back of this book.

The worktext opens with a Pre-Assessment to help identify areas of focus. It concludes with a Post-Assessment to identify concepts that may need reinforcement.

The combination of the interactive activities in the online course and the pencil-and-paper practice in the worktext enhances the student's ability to learn math concepts. It provides the optimal learning environment for a subject that requires repetition and multiple methods of practice in order to internalize concepts. Best of all, students can work through the material at a pace with which they are comfortable. We hope this course empowers the reader with the skills and confidence needed to realize their full potential in the healthcare industry.

Contents

BASIC MATH FOR HEALTH PROFESSIONALS

Pre-Assessment

Answer the following questions. Answers to the Pre-Assessment are found in the back of your workbook.

1. Which of the following is a whole number?

$$\left\{ 7, \frac{1}{2}, 0.12 \right\}$$

2. Which of the following is the larger number?

   5   or   −15

3. What is the absolute value of 7?

4. What is the absolute value of −7|?

5. Which is the larger number?

   1.001678   or   100.1678

6. What number does the Roman Numeral represent VIII?

7. What number does the Roman Numeral represent XIV?

8. What would be the Roman Numeral for the number 26?

9. What number is in the ones place of 715.41?

10. What number is in the tenth place of 68.742?

Solve for the following equations.

11. $101 + 54$

12. $191 + 44 + 16$

13. $117 - 64$

14. $820.75 + 130.15$

15. $4.2 - 0.9 - 1.5$

16. 32×7

17. $416 \times 5 \times 2$

18. 1.8×0.21

19. $126 \div 3$

1

20. $294 \div 1.4$

21. $(15 \div 3) + 110$

22. $21 \times 3 + (13 \times 3)$

23. Which of the following is the larger number?

$\frac{1}{8}$ or $\frac{5}{8}$

24. Convert $\frac{16}{3}$ to a mixed number.

25. Convert $\frac{9}{5}$ to a mixed number.

26. Convert $4\frac{2}{5}$ to an improper fraction.

27. Reduce $\frac{20}{100}$ to the lowest term

28. Reduce $\frac{44}{220}$ to the lowest term.

Solve for the following equations. Reduce to the lowest term.

29. $\frac{3}{4} + \frac{4}{5}$

30. $4\frac{1}{3} + \frac{7}{12}$

31. $\frac{7}{10} - \frac{9}{20}$

32. $9\frac{1}{3} - 6\frac{3}{4}$

33. $\frac{2}{3} \times \frac{3}{5}$

34. $1\frac{4}{5} \times \frac{1}{2}$

35. $\frac{9}{10} \div \frac{1}{5}$

36. $2\frac{7}{10} \div \frac{3}{4}$

37. Convert 0.15 to a fraction and to the lowest term.

38. Convert 7.2 to a fraction and to the lowest term.

39. Round 1.71256 to the nearest thousandth place.

40. Round 80.198 to the nearest tenth place.

41. Convert 65.5% into a decimal.

42. Convert 125% into a fraction.

43. Convert 4:20 to a fraction and to the lowest term.

44. Convert 11:4 to a fraction and to the lowest term.

45. Solve for *x*.

$$\frac{2}{5} = \frac{x}{10}$$

46. Solve for x.

$$\frac{x}{20} = \frac{4}{5}$$

47. Solve for *x*.

$$x : 15 = 3 : 5$$

48. A car you want to buy is $5,200. The dealership is offering a discount of 8%. How much will this car cost after the discount?

49. A teaspoon of salt is added to every 2 cups of water. How many teaspoons would you add for 6 cups of water?

50. You want to buy pizza for 10 of your friends. You think each person will have 3 slices each. There are 8 slices in a pizza. How many pizzas should you buy?

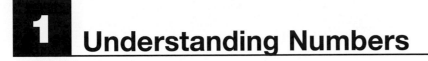

1 Understanding Numbers

WHOLE NUMBERS, PLACE VALUES, INTEGERS, AND ABSOLUTE VALUES

Practice Exercise 1A

Return to Module 1 Screen 1.6 of the Online Course for step-by-step solutions.

Solve for the following problems.

1. Which of the following is a whole number?
   A. −14
   B. 0
   C. 14
   D. All the above

2. Which of the following is an integer?
   A. 0
   B. 14
   C. −14
   D. All the above

3. What is the absolute value of 6?

4. List the place value of the following number: −215

5. List the place value of the following number: −6174

Practice Drills 1A

Answers to Practice Drills are found in the back of your workbook.

Answer the following questions. Which of the following is a whole number?

1. $-2, \dfrac{1}{2}, 2$

2. 0, −2.12, 2.12

3. 0.4, 718986, $\dfrac{4}{10}$

4. 11, −11, + 0.11

5. 0.10, 1.10, 10

For the following numbers, Identify the place value of the circled number.

6. ⑤1

7. 51⓪

8. 17⑤,850

9. 2,⑤00,875

10. 1②,463,5012

Identify the integer.

11. $-17, 0.17, \dfrac{1}{7}$

12. $1.5, 1000.01, 0$

13. 130 pounds weight loss

14. thermometer shows 99 °F

15. 5 degrees below zero

What is the opposite of each integer?

16. -4

17. 515

18. $+11$

19. -135

20. 0

Identify the number in each of the following sentences.

21. A six-pack of beer

22. A box of 50 gloves

23. A medium-sized pizza has eight slices of pizza

24. A large-sized pizza has twelve slices of pizza

25. The temperature in Toledo in wintertime can be as low as 5 degrees below freezing

26. A typical carton of eggs

27. A pair of socks

28. Number of fingers

29. Number of tires on a car

30. A dozen roses

ROMAN NUMERALS

Practice Exercise 1B
Convert the following Arabic numbers to Roman numerals. Return to Module 1 Screen 2.5 of the Online Course for step-by-step solutions.

1. 7

2. 12

3. 15

4. 30

5. 19

Practice Drills 1B
Convert the following numerals to Arabic or Roman numerals.
Answers to Practice Drills are found in the back of your workbook.

1. XIII

2. XV

3. xxxiii

4. IV

5. XXII

6. xxiv

7. xxii

8. XVI

9. XXXVII

10. XXIX

11. 3

12. 5

13. 9

14. 17

15. 27

16. 12

17. 39

18. 14

19. 34

20. 28

21. 33

7

22. 19

23. 10

24. 12

25. 21

26. 36

27. 31

28. 20

29. 27

30. 15

31. XXII

32. XVI

33. III

34. XXVIII

35. XIV

36. VIII

37. XIX

38. VII

39. XIV

40. XXXII

USING LARGER ROMAN NUMERALS

Practice Exercise 1C

Convert the following Roman numerals to Arabic numbers. Return to Module 1 Screen 2.7 of the Online Course for step-by-step solutions.

1. XC

2. LV

3. XVII

4. XLII

5. LXIV

Practice Drills 1C

Convert the following numerals to Arabic or Roman numerals.
Answers to Practice Drills are found in the back of your workbook.

1. 40

2. 90

3. 400

4. 120

5. 950

6. 58

7. 240

8. 514

9. 404

10. 2,150

11. LI

12. CX

13. CXV1

14. LV

15. MI

16. CDXCIX

17. CMXCIX

18. LXXXIX

19. XCIX

20. CDLXXIV

21. LXXXII

22. CI

23. 23.DCCI

24. LIV

25. LXVI

26. LXXIII

27. XC

28. MII

29. DXXXV

30. XLIX

31. 433

32. 530

33. 50

34. 93

35. 550

36. LXVIII

37. MD

38. DCII

39. CDLVI

40. CCCXIII

REVIEW EXERCISES

Using the methods in this chapter, solve for the following problems. Return to the online course to review any content. Answers to Review Exercises are found in the back of your workbook.

1. What is the place value for 7 in the number 17?

2. What is the place value for 4 in the number 482?

3. What is the place value for 3 in the number 7,368?

4. What is the place value for 2 in the number 1,512?

5. What is the place value for 2 in the number 7,125,980?

6. What is the place value for 8 in the number 8,242,012?

7. $|\,17\,| = ?$

8. $|\,{-44}\,| = ?$

9. $|\,0\,| = ?$

10. $|\,{+3,425}\,| = ?$

11. Which of the following is a whole number?
    A. 1.2
    B. 5
    C. −7
    D. 0.12

12. Which of the following is a whole number?
    A. $\frac{3}{8}$
    B. 4.15
    C. $-\frac{1}{3}$
    D. 0

13. Which of the following is a positive integer?
    A. 1.2
    B. 5
    C. −7
    D. 0

14. Which of the following is a negative integer?
    A. 1.2
    B. 5
    C. −7
    D. 0

15. Which of the following is NOT an integer?
    A. 1.2
    B. 5
    C. −7
    D. 0

16. Which of the following is an integer?
    A. +152
    B. 0.152
    C. $\frac{3}{8}$
    D. $-\frac{3}{8}$

Convert the Roman numerals to Arabic numerals.

17. XI

18. IX

19. LI

20. MD

21. XVII

22. XXXIII

23. XLIX

24. XXXVIII

25. XXXIV

26. CXXX

27. CLV

28. CLXII

29. CXLII

30. LXXIX

31. XCVII

32. CLIII

33. LXVII

Convert the Arabic numerals to Roman numerals.

34. 8

35. 12

36. 19

37. 43

38. 28

39. 15

40. 54

41. 38

42. 90

43. 86

44. 890

45. 153

46. 742

47. 738

48. 672

49. 556

50. 974

2 Basic Addition and Subtraction

ADDITION

Practice Exercise 2A

Solve for the following problems. Return to Module 2 Screen 1.8 of the Online Course for step-by-step solutions.

1. 194 + 67

2. 711 + 358

3. 999 + 1215

4. 4871 + 6712

5. 213 + 565 + 489

Practice Drills 2A

Answers to Practice Drills are found in the back of your workbook.

Solve for the following problems.

1. 13 + 2

2. 16 + 4

3. 78 + 5

4. 89 + 2

5. 55 + 24

6. 74 + 81

7. 155 + 10

8. 612 + 18

9. 419 + 63

10. 234 + 44

11. 200 + 60 + 5

12. 703 + 25 + 7

13. 713 + 38 + 7

14. 123 + 777

15. 567 + 867

13

16. 712 + 138

17. 602 + 331 + 47

18. 1,433 + 9,829

19. 333 + 45 + 87 + 1,212

20. 4,531 + 2,551 + 91 + 8

21. 567 + 867 + 1,001

22. 321 + 123 + 111

23. 987 + 1,100 + 113

24. 4,572 + 7,255

25. Add 2,365 and 4,111.

26. Add 3,127 and 1,652.

27. Add 37,685 and 24,739.

28. Add 67,459 and 56,678.

29. What is the sum of 4373, 4191, and 3127?

30. Find the sum of 583497, 275634, and 13205.

31. Andie has 20 pieces of chocolate and 30 pieces of taffy. How many pieces of candy does she have?

32. Vicky has 14 shells and found 72 more on the beach. How many shells does she have?

33. A school has 458 boys and 524 girls. How many attend the school?

34. You have $325 and then received $725. How much money do you have?

35. A family is looking to take two vacations this year. The first vacation costs $1,185. The second vacation costs $3,450. How much will be the costs of both trips?

36. In a city, there are 60,345 men, 69,252 women and 33,258 children. What is the total population of the city?

37. A concert had the following attendees over the course of several days: 5,096 and 4,901. How many people attended?

38. Celia is an avid marathon runner. In one year, she ran 1,300 miles. The second year, she ran 1,450 miles, and the next year she ran 1,520 miles. How many miles did she run over these years?

39. A store sold 7,250 crates of milk for the past two years. This year, it will sell 4,115 crates. How many crates of milk was sold in the last 3 years?

40. The population in Seattle in 2019 was 3,433,000 people. The city was projected to grow by 56,000 by 2021. What is the population in 2021?

SUBTRACTION

Practice Exercise 2B

Solve for the following problems. Return to Module 2 Screen 2.6 of the Online Course for step-by-step solutions.

1. 67 – 56

2. 248 – 52

3. 898 – 499

4. 765 – 88

5. 547 – 269

Practice Drills 2B

Answers to Practice Drills are found in the back of your workbook.

Solve for the following problems.

1. 17 – 10

2. 18 – 3

3. 29 – 12

4. 35 – 8

5. 105 – 9

6. 514 – 8

7. 75 – 23

8. 92 – 81

9. 49 – 17

10. 123 – 97

11. 67 – 56

12. 212 – 10

13. 289 – 54

14. 4,547 – 2,298

15. 657 – 259

16. 148 – 52

17. 6,212 – 1,978

18. 5,841 – 2,237

19. 4,547 − 2,289 − 200

20. 1,150 − 712 − 515

21. 765 − 731

22. 637 − 137

23. 557 − 269

24. 765 − 89

25. 898 − 949

26. 1857 − 949

27. 375 − 368 − 15

28. 657 − 259 − 67

29. 5,840 − 2,237 − 52

30. 4,152 − 654 − 499

31. Subtract 39 from 78.

32. Subtract 189 from 638.

33. Solve for 74,834 − 38,915.

34. Subtract 39,507 − 27,386.

35. What is the difference of 3867 and 1298?

36. There are 71 coins in a purse. You take out 25 coins. How many are left?

37. A raffle sells 73 tickets and started out with 210. How many tickets are left?

38. The population of Toledo, Ohio in 2012 was 287,487. In 2022, the population was 266,524. How many people left the city?

39. Subtract 4,358 from the sum of 5,632 and 1,324.

40. Subtract 17,583 from the sum of 31,101 and 7,984.

REVIEW EXERCISES

Using the methods in this chapter, solve for the following problems. Return to the online course to review any content. Answers to Review Exercises are found in the back of your workbook.

1. 4 + 3

2. 7 + 9

3. $17 - 5$

4. $89 - 11$

5. $67 - 56$

6. $5 + 8 + 4 + 7$

7. $1 + 5 + 9 + 2$

8. $51 + 23$

9. $75 + 15$

10. $46 + 18$

11. $43 + 28$

12. $450 + 82$

13. $289 + 17$

14. $194 + 67$

15. $709 + 49$

16. $212 - 10$

17. $289 - 54$

18. $475 - 34$

19. $358 - 65$

20. $148 - 52$

21. $657 - 259$

22. $4,801 - 898$

23. $4,547 - 2,298$

24. $1,236 - 979$

25. $10,300 - 479$

26. $6,212 - 1,978$

27. $1,556 + 123$

28. $24,578 + 9,075$

29. $56 + 811 + 9$

30. 165 + 76 + 214

31. 968 + 19 + 45

32. 2,003 + 2,851 + 91

33. 443 + 134 + 2,087

34. 297 + 90 + 105 + 6

35. 2,102 + 3 + 297 + 90

36. 11 + 34 + 86 + 357

37. 1,733 + 57 + 213 + 212

38. 134 + 443 + 2,087 + 555

39. 5,841 − 2,237

40. 14,713 − 4,347

41. 82,999 − 22,476

42. 115,789 − 56,117

43. 210,810 − 114,561

44. 4,547 − 2,289 − 200

45. 1,150 − 712 − 515

46. 167 + 99 − 56

47. 6,212 − 1,989 + 117

48. 74,939 + 560 − 717

49. 54,856 − 99 − 14,751 + 2,140

50. 11,190 + 615 + 444 − 25,145

3 Basic Multiplication and Division

BASIC MULTIPLICATION

Practice Exercise 3A

Solve for the following problems using the following methods:

- Repeat a number and then add

- Use the multiplication table

Return to Module 3 Screen 1.5 of the Online Course for step-by-step solutions.

1. What is two times five?

2. What is three times six?

3. What is seven times four?

Practice Drills 3A

Write the following as a multiplication problem.
Answers to Practice Drills are found in the back of your workbook.

1. $2 + 2 + 2$

2. $4 + 4$

3. $1 + 1 + 1 + 1 + 1$

4. $6 + 6 + 6 + 6$

5. $8 + 8 + 8$

6. $3 + 3 + 3 + 3$

7. $10 + 10 + 10 + 10$

Solve for the following problems.

8. 2×3

9. 4×2

10. 1×5

11. 6×4

12. 8×3

13. 3×4

14. 10×4

15. 2×14

16. 11×8

17. 70×9

18. 12×4

19. 44×2

20. 12×3

21. 13×3

22. 5×12

23. 3×6

24. 8×2

25. 5×3

26. 2×7

27. 5×6

28. 4×11

29. 3×12

30. 9×10

31. 9×3

32. 11×11

33. 4×12

34. 10×2

35. 7×8

36. There are 5 pieces of candy in 2 boxes. How many total pieces of candy do you have?

37. You are having a party and want to order pizza. Each person should have 2 slices of pizza and there are 8 people. How many slices should you order?

38. Sonia is packing for a trip. She will be gone for 7 days and wants to make sure she has two pairs of socks for each day. How many pairs of socks should she pack?

39. Will wants to ship as many books as possible in 10 boxes. Each box can fit 10 books. How many books can he ship?

40. A pharmacy technician is restocking the pill cabinet. There are 7 shelves, and 12 pill bottles can be placed on each shelf. How many pill bottles can be restocked?

41. A medical office is trying to determine how many patients it can see in 5 days. The office manager determines that 12 patients can be seen each day. How many patients can be seen?

MULTIPLYING WITH THE COLUMN METHOD

Practice Exercise 3B

Solve for the following problems. Return to Module 3 Screen 1.7 of the Online Course for solutions.

1. 12×7

2. 30×3

3. 62×4

4. 321×2

5. 210×3

Practice Drills 3B

Answers to Practice Drills are found in the back of your workbook.

Solve for the following problems.

1. 13×3

2. 10×5

3. 11×7

4. 60×3

5. 70×9

6. 20×7

7. 51×8

8. 50×5

9. 610×5

10. 187×3

11. 321×4

12. 222×3

13. 600×4

14. 411×3

Module **3** Basic Multiplication and Division

15. 533×2

16. $1,422 \times 2$

17. $8,322 \times 3$

18. $4,012 \times 4$

19. $2,101 \times 7$

20. $40,414 \times 2$

21. 123×5

22. 279×7

23. 928×8

24. 351×6

25. 542×3

26. 642×8

27. 439×5

28. 681×7

29. 472×4

30. 567×3

31. $1,298 \times 6$

32. $9,992 \times 5$

33. $3,487 \times 8$

34. $4,756 \times 3$

35. 765×8

36. $13,612 \times 9$

37. $7,819 \times 4$

38. $12,850 \times 7$

39. $91,615 \times 8$

40. $77,227 \times 9$

MULTIPLICATION WITH CARRY OVER

Practice Exercise 3C

Solve for the following problems. Return to Module 3 Screen 1.9 of the Online Course for step-by-step solutions.

1. 11×8

2. 60×3

3. 25×12

4. 750×22

5. $2,456 \times 111$

Practice Drills 3C

Answers to Practice Drills are found in the back of your workbook.

Solve for the following problems.

1. 16×3

2. 12×8

3. 87×5

4. 48×12

5. 927×35

6. 512×21

7. 72×13

8. 803×17

9. 346×12

10. 189×27

11. 178×23

12. $1,306 \times 18$

13. $1,020 \times 95$

14. $5,791 \times 16$

15. $9,004 \times 72$

16. $2,346 \times 15$

17. $8,753 \times 65$

18. $74,943 \times 27$

23

19. $12{,}564 \times 18$

20. $46{,}882 \times 175$

21. 838×3

22. 118×6

23. 163×2

24. 271×4

25. 841×5

26. 318×2

27. 233×8

28. 339×9

29. 947×8

30. 143×6

31. $1{,}125 \times 5$

32. $1{,}406 \times 3$

33. $3{,}271 \times 4$

34. $6{,}374 \times 5$

35. $28{,}470 \times 4$

36. $14{,}932 \times 2$

37. $92{,}745 \times 6$

38. $74{,}516 \times 8$

39. $82{,}605 \times 9$

40. $21{,}315 \times 5$

LONG DIVISION

Practice Exercise 3D

Solve for the following problems. Return to Module 3 Screen 2.5 of the Online Course for step-by-step solutions.

1. $81 \div 3$

2. $564 \div 6$

3. $4\overline{)12345}$

24

4. $10\overline{)8743}$

5. $15\overline{)154560}$

Practice Drills 3D

Answers to Practice Drills are found in the back of your workbook.

Solve for the following problems.

1. 20 divided by 2

2. 25 divided by 5

3. 16 divided by 4

4. 56 divided by 8

5. 75 divided by 15

6. 25 divided by 6

7. 37 divided by 3

8. $932 \div 8$

9. $5,860 \div 14$

10. $750 \div 100$

11. $655 \div 5$

12. $843 \div 82$

13. $984 \div 60$

14. $754 \div 65$

15. $\dfrac{25}{20}$

16. $\dfrac{23}{7}$

17. $\dfrac{23}{4}$

18. $\dfrac{907}{12}$

19. $\dfrac{235}{9}$

20. $\dfrac{1250}{50}$

21. $7,543 \div 5$

22. $3,874 \div 4$

23. 8,507 ÷ 6

24. 1,991 ÷ 8

25. 4,123 ÷ 3

26. 8,862 ÷ 8

27. 6,276 ÷ 7

28. 6,589 ÷ 4

29. 1,959 ÷ 3

30. 7,367 ÷ 2

31. 2,153 ÷ 9

32. 8,592 ÷ 6

33. 4,356 ÷ 9

34. 2,435 ÷ 9

35. 3,692 ÷ 4

36. 1,000 ÷ 8

37. 3,246 ÷ 6

38. 13,620 ÷ 3

39. 89,100 ÷ 5

40. 55,912 ÷ 7

ORDER OF OPERATIONS

Practice Exercise 3E

Solve for the following problems. Return to Module 3 Screen 3.3 of the Online Course for step-by-step solutions.

1. $2 \times (3 + 4)$

2. $10(48 \div 2)$

3. $48 \div 2 (9 + 3)$

4. $(48 \div 2)9 + 3$

5. $600 \div (3 \times 8 + 6) - 10$

Practice Drills 3E

Answers to Practice Drills are found in the back of your workbook.

Solve for the following problems.

1. $7 \times 3 + 5$

2. $37 - 2 \times 2$

3. $4 + 9 \times 5$

4. $95 - 2 \times 3$

5. $8 + 3 \times 5$

6. $2 \times (4 + 8)$

7. $93 - (2 \times 7)$

8. $85 - (2 \times 5)$

9. $(10 - 1)\,4$

10. $(3 + 4)\,8$

11. $10 + (2 \times 4) \div 2$

12. $(2 + 3)(1 + 2)$

13. $(104) - 32 \div 4$

14. $(11)5 \times 3 - 10$

15. $125 - (20 \div 4)$

16. $42 + (6 \times 4) \div 2$

17. $96 \div 2(1 + 2)$

18. $(1 \times 5 + 27) - 32 \div 4$

19. $8 + 2 \times 5(8)$

20. $96 \div 3 + (20)3$

21. $15 \times 60 \div 20$

22. $2 \times 50 \div 10$

23. $4 \times 25 \div 5$

24. $9 \times 6 \div 8 + 11$

25. $77 \div (3 + 4)$

26. $5 \times (13 - 4)$

Module **3** **Basic Multiplication and Division**

27. $6 + 24 \div (5 + 1)$

28. $(8 + 10) \times (7\text{-}6)$

29. $33 - (3 \times 6 - 9)$

30. $84 \div 7 \times (9 + 11)$

31. $8 + (66 \div 6 \times 8) + 11 - 3$

32. $189 \div (12 + 9)$

33. $3 + 30 \div (4 + 2)$

34. $36 \div 6 \times (5 + 10)$

35. $3 + (44 \div 4 \times 12) + 9 - 11$

36. $2 + 50 \div (4 + 6)$

37. $21 - (3 \times 0 - 11)$

38. $81 \div 9 \times (9 + 12)$

39. $2 + (48 \div 4 \times 8) + 3 - 2$

40. $(36 \div 4 \times 5) + 1 - 4$

REVIEW EXERCISES

Using the methods in this chapter, solve for the following problems. Return to the online course to review any content. Answers to Review Exercises are found in the back of your workbook.

1. 7 times 5

2. 4 times 6

3. 11 times 3

4. 16 times 4

5. 1×5

6. 4×7

7. 8×6

8. $3 \times 3 \times 2$

9. $5 \times 9 \times 0$

10. 15×4

11. $6 \times 6 \times 3$

12. $14 \times 1 \times 4$

13. $7 \times 11 \times 2$

14. 12×7

15. 47×20

16. $1,000 \times 100$

17. 222×12

18. 463×13

19. $1,786 \times 10$

20. 828×4

21. $2,211 \times 11$

22. $100 \times 10 \times 8$

23. $15 \times 4 \times 16 \times 2$

24. $1,149 \times 45$

25. $3,133 \times 52$

26. $925 \times 46 \times 2$

27. 470×491

28. $8,411 \times 825$

29. $2,771 \times 4,958$

30. $1,320 \times 22 \times 12$

31. 16 divided by 4

32. 5 divided by 0

33. 15 divided by 3

34. $\dfrac{24}{6}$

35. $\dfrac{165}{15}$

36. $75 \div 15$

37. $844 \div 4$

38. $655 \div 5$

39. $480 \div 30$

40. $1,040 \div 65$

41. $6 \div 3 \times 2$

42. $14 + 28 \div 4$

43. $(3 + 4)(8 + 4)$

44. $(3 + 4) + (8 + 4)$

45. $40 - (4 + 6) \div 2 + 3$

46. $77 - (1 + 4 - 2)2$

47. $150 \div (6 + 3 \times 8) - 5$

48. $(36 - 6) \div (12 + 3)$

49. $5 \times 8 + 6 \div 6 - 12 \times 2$

50. $(36 - 3 \times 4) \div (15 - 9 \div 3)$

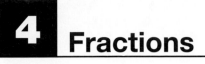

Fractions

TYPES OF FRACTIONS

Practice Exercise 4A

Identify the types of fractions as proper, improper, or mixed. Return to Module 4 Screen 1.5 of the Online Course for solutions.

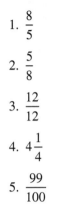

1. $\dfrac{8}{5}$

2. $\dfrac{5}{8}$

3. $\dfrac{12}{12}$

4. $4\dfrac{1}{4}$

5. $\dfrac{99}{100}$

Practice Drills 4A

Identify the types of fractions as proper, improper, or mixed. Answers to Practice Drills are found in the back of your workbook.

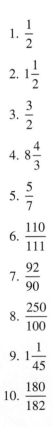

1. $\dfrac{1}{2}$

2. $1\dfrac{1}{2}$

3. $\dfrac{3}{2}$

4. $8\dfrac{4}{3}$

5. $\dfrac{5}{7}$

6. $\dfrac{110}{111}$

7. $\dfrac{92}{90}$

8. $\dfrac{250}{100}$

9. $1\dfrac{1}{45}$

10. $\dfrac{180}{182}$

11. $\dfrac{7}{12}$

12. $2\dfrac{2}{5}$

13. $\dfrac{12}{5}$

14. $\dfrac{23}{7}$

15. $3\dfrac{2}{7}$

16. $\dfrac{15}{16}$

17. $\dfrac{75}{4}$

18. $\dfrac{87}{88}$

19. $4\dfrac{5}{9}$

20. $\dfrac{1000}{1001}$

21. $\dfrac{13}{15}$

22. $\dfrac{99}{55}$

23. $\dfrac{590}{589}$

24. $21\dfrac{1}{3}$

25. $\dfrac{5}{17}$

26. $\dfrac{17}{5}$

27. $3\dfrac{2}{5}$

28. $\dfrac{7}{213}$

29. $30\dfrac{3}{7}$

30. $\dfrac{29}{23}$

31. $\dfrac{123}{273}$

32. $2\dfrac{111}{100}$

32

33. $\dfrac{100}{111}$

34. $\dfrac{13}{52}$

35. $\dfrac{25}{35}$

36. $\dfrac{64}{24}$

37. $3\dfrac{8}{24}$

38. $\dfrac{49}{65}$

39. $\dfrac{20}{200}$

40. $100\dfrac{6}{5}$

CONVERTING FRACTIONS

Practice Exercise 4B

Convert the following numbers to either a mixed number or improper fraction. Return to Module 4 Screen 2.6 of the Online Course for solutions.

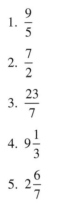

1. $\dfrac{9}{5}$

2. $\dfrac{7}{2}$

3. $\dfrac{23}{7}$

4. $9\dfrac{1}{3}$

5. $2\dfrac{6}{7}$

Practice Drills 4B

Convert the following numbers to either a mixed number or improper fraction. Answers to Practice Drills are found in the back of your workbook.

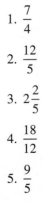

1. $\dfrac{7}{4}$

2. $\dfrac{12}{5}$

3. $2\dfrac{2}{5}$

4. $\dfrac{18}{12}$

5. $\dfrac{9}{5}$

6. $\dfrac{12}{12}$

7. $5\dfrac{3}{4}$

8. $3\dfrac{7}{12}$

9. $2\dfrac{6}{7}$

10. $\dfrac{16}{15}$

11. $\dfrac{56}{14}$

12. $\dfrac{38}{3}$

13. $1\dfrac{15}{16}$

14. $\dfrac{25}{20}$

15. $\dfrac{88}{33}$

16. $9\dfrac{1}{3}$

17. $2\dfrac{4}{19}$

18. $\dfrac{75}{4}$

19. $\dfrac{144}{13}$

20. $7\dfrac{12}{13}$

21. $1\dfrac{13}{15}$

22. $\dfrac{99}{55}$

23. $\dfrac{590}{589}$

24. $21\dfrac{1}{3}$

25. $3\dfrac{5}{17}$

26. $\dfrac{17}{5}$

27. $3\dfrac{2}{5}$

34

28. $1\dfrac{7}{213}$

29. $30\dfrac{3}{7}$

30. $\dfrac{29}{23}$

31. $10\dfrac{123}{273}$

32. $2\dfrac{111}{100}$

33. $4\dfrac{100}{111}$

34. $5\dfrac{13}{52}$

35. $\dfrac{35}{25}$

36. $\dfrac{64}{24}$

37. $3\dfrac{8}{24}$

38. $\dfrac{65}{49}$

39. $\dfrac{201}{20}$

40. $100\dfrac{6}{5}$

Practice Exercise 4C

Reduce the following fractions to their lowest term. Return to Module 4 Screen 2.11 of the Online Course for solutions.

1. $\dfrac{16}{20}$

2. $\dfrac{3}{36}$

3. $\dfrac{33}{55}$

4. $\dfrac{21}{27}$

5. $\dfrac{14}{56}$

Practice Drills 4C

Reduce the following fractions to their lowest term. Answers to Practice Drills are found in the back of your workbook.

1. $\dfrac{3}{6}$

2. $\dfrac{4}{8}$

3. $\dfrac{5}{20}$

4. $\dfrac{15}{75}$

5. $\dfrac{8}{72}$

6. $\dfrac{4}{3}$

7. $\dfrac{16}{15}$

8. $\dfrac{7}{3}$

9. $\dfrac{20}{25}$

10. $\dfrac{33}{88}$

11. $\dfrac{42}{48}$

12. $\dfrac{38}{12}$

13. $\dfrac{41}{9}$

14. $\dfrac{39}{12}$

15. $\dfrac{42}{19}$

16. $\dfrac{72}{144}$

17. $\dfrac{75}{4}$

18. $\dfrac{94}{8}$

19. $\dfrac{144}{33}$

20. $\dfrac{92}{44}$

21. $\dfrac{15}{18}$

22. $\dfrac{14}{42}$

23. $\dfrac{30}{35}$

24. $\dfrac{56}{22}$

25. $\dfrac{27}{42}$

26. $\dfrac{28}{11}$

27. $\dfrac{18}{32}$

28. $\dfrac{80}{30}$

29. $\dfrac{16}{36}$

30. $\dfrac{49}{25}$

31. $\dfrac{125}{15}$

32. $\dfrac{139}{8}$

33. $\dfrac{279}{16}$

34. $\dfrac{56}{49}$

35. $2\dfrac{81}{21}$

36. $7\dfrac{9}{7}$

37. $10\dfrac{54}{12}$

38. $14\dfrac{52}{39}$

39. $\dfrac{600}{24}$

40. $51\dfrac{100}{75}$

ADDING AND SUBTRACTING FRACTIONS

Practice Exercise 4D

Solve for the following equations and reduce to the lowest term. Return to Module 4 Screen 3.4 of the Online Course for solutions.

1. $\dfrac{2}{3}+\dfrac{7}{9}$

2. $1\frac{1}{10}+\frac{3}{5}$

3. $1\frac{3}{8}-\frac{1}{2}$

4. $2\frac{3}{4}+1\frac{2}{3}$

5. $\frac{2}{3}+\frac{7}{9}+2\frac{2}{5}$

Practice Drills 4D

Solve for the following equations and reduce to the lowest term. Answers to Practice Drills are found in the back of your workbook.

1. $\frac{1}{2}+\frac{1}{2}$

   2. $\frac{4}{5}+\frac{2}{5}$

2. $\frac{3}{5}+\frac{1}{5}$

3. $\frac{7}{15}+\frac{3}{15}$

4. $\frac{2}{7}+\frac{5}{7}$

5. $\frac{1}{8}+\frac{3}{8}+\frac{5}{8}$

6. $\frac{8}{15}-\frac{7}{15}$

7. $\frac{16}{17}-\frac{10}{17}$

8. $\frac{35}{94}-\frac{9}{94}-\frac{11}{94}$

9. $\frac{2}{7}+\frac{2}{3}$

10. $\frac{12}{21}-\frac{3}{7}$

11. $\frac{5}{6}+\frac{3}{4}$

12. $\frac{13}{33}+\frac{1}{11}+\frac{2}{11}$

13. $4\frac{2}{3}+\frac{2}{3}$

14. $\frac{2}{3}+3\frac{5}{9}$

15. $3\frac{3}{4}-1\frac{2}{5}$

16. $1\dfrac{9}{22}-\dfrac{15}{11}$

17. $2\dfrac{20}{21}-\dfrac{3}{7}$

18. $1\dfrac{7}{8}+\dfrac{2}{13}$

19. $3\dfrac{5}{9}-\dfrac{2}{3}+\dfrac{3}{4}$

20. $1\dfrac{1}{3}+5\dfrac{2}{5}-\dfrac{7}{9}$

21. $5\dfrac{3}{8}+2\dfrac{1}{4}$

22. $\dfrac{2}{3}+\dfrac{8}{9}$

23. $\dfrac{5}{6}+\dfrac{7}{12}$

24. $\dfrac{40}{100}+\dfrac{3}{5}$

25. $\dfrac{7}{11}+\dfrac{4}{10}$

26. $4\dfrac{1}{4}+\dfrac{11}{12}$

27. $\dfrac{7}{3}+\dfrac{17}{6}$

28. $\dfrac{41}{30}+\dfrac{11}{10}$

29. $1\dfrac{4}{21}+1\dfrac{5}{7}$

30. $1\dfrac{4}{5}+\dfrac{37}{30}$

31. $3\dfrac{2}{3}+1\dfrac{5}{18}$

32. $\dfrac{13}{10}+2\dfrac{1}{3}$

33. $\dfrac{28}{10}+1\dfrac{9}{10}$

34. $1\dfrac{6}{7}+1\dfrac{1}{5}$

35. $1\dfrac{5}{8}+2\dfrac{1}{10}$

36. $\dfrac{14}{3}+3\dfrac{2}{5}$

37. $1\dfrac{5}{9}+1\dfrac{2}{5}$

38. $3\frac{1}{2}+1\frac{5}{8}$

39. $1\frac{1}{7}+2\frac{1}{4}$

40. $1\frac{5}{7}+2\frac{1}{5}$

MULTIPLYING FRACTIONS

Practice Exercise 4E

Multiply the following fractions and reduce to the lowest term. Return to Module 4 Screen 4.2 of the Online Course for solutions.

1. $\frac{5}{7}\times\frac{1}{3}$

2. $\frac{9}{10}\times\frac{3}{10}$

3. $\frac{4}{5}\times4\frac{1}{2}$

4. $5\frac{5}{8}\times2\frac{1}{3}$

5. $\frac{1}{3}\times\frac{3}{4}\times3\frac{1}{2}$

Practice Drills 4E

Multiply the following fractions and reduce to the lowest term. Answers to Practice Drills are found in the back of your workbook.

1. $\frac{1}{2}\times\frac{2}{5}$

2. $\frac{3}{4}\times\frac{1}{4}$

3. $\frac{4}{5}\times\frac{1}{4}$

4. $\frac{2}{3}\times\frac{1}{3}$

5. $\frac{3}{8}\times\frac{3}{4}$

6. $\frac{1}{4}\times5$

7. $\frac{2}{6}\times6$

8. $\frac{3}{8}\times2$

9. $\frac{5}{12}\times2$

10. $2\frac{2}{5}\times\frac{4}{5}$

11. $\dfrac{3}{4} \times 4\dfrac{7}{12}$

12. $4\dfrac{1}{2} \times \dfrac{1}{6}$

13. $\dfrac{1}{3} \times 8\dfrac{2}{3}$

14. $2\dfrac{1}{3} \times 4\dfrac{1}{2}$

15. $\dfrac{1}{5} \times \dfrac{3}{4} \times \dfrac{4}{9} \times \dfrac{1}{7}$

16. $\dfrac{1}{7} \times \dfrac{5}{11} \times 3\dfrac{1}{2} \times 1\dfrac{2}{7}$

17. $1\dfrac{3}{7} \times 1\dfrac{1}{4} \times \dfrac{9}{10} \times \dfrac{1}{3}$

18. $\dfrac{1}{4} \times \dfrac{5}{7} \times 1\dfrac{3}{8} \times \dfrac{7}{8}$

19. $\dfrac{9}{11} \times 1\dfrac{3}{7} \times 7\dfrac{1}{2} \times \dfrac{3}{4}$

20. $2\dfrac{1}{4} \times 5\dfrac{1}{2} \times 2\dfrac{1}{2} \times 1\dfrac{1}{4}$

21. $1\dfrac{1}{2} \times 4\dfrac{4}{7}$

22. $5 \times \dfrac{8}{10}$

23. $3\dfrac{2}{5} \times 3$

24. $6\dfrac{1}{2} \times 3\dfrac{1}{3}$

25. $4\dfrac{1}{3} \times 3$

26. $1\dfrac{4}{7} \times \dfrac{3}{2}$

27. $3\dfrac{1}{4} \times 5$

28. $2\dfrac{3}{5} \times \dfrac{3}{4}$

29. $1\dfrac{1}{8} \times 2\dfrac{1}{5}$

30. $2\dfrac{1}{4} \times \dfrac{7}{10}$

31. $1\dfrac{6}{7} \times \dfrac{5}{6}$

32. $4 \times 2\dfrac{2}{3}$

33. $1\dfrac{7}{10} \times \dfrac{3}{8}$

34. $5\dfrac{1}{2} \times 1\dfrac{3}{4}$

35. $4\dfrac{2}{3} \times \dfrac{5}{12}$

36. $4\dfrac{1}{5} \times 2\dfrac{2}{9}$

37. $2\dfrac{5}{9} \times \dfrac{2}{5}$

38. $2\dfrac{3}{5} \times \dfrac{4}{9}$

39. $5\dfrac{1}{3} \times 1\dfrac{1}{2}$

40. $\dfrac{4}{7} \times 4\dfrac{1}{6}$

DIVIDING FRACTIONS

Practice Exercise 4F

Solve for the following problems and reduce to the lowest term. Return to Module 4 Screen 4.5 of the Online Course for solutions.

1. $\dfrac{4}{5} \div \dfrac{1}{4}$

2. $4\dfrac{1}{2} \div 2\dfrac{1}{3}$

3. $3\dfrac{3}{5} \div 2\dfrac{3}{10}$

4. $1\dfrac{1}{3} \div \dfrac{1}{8}$

5. $9\dfrac{1}{5} \div 2$

Practice Drills 4F

Solve for the following problems and reduce to the lowest term. Answers to Practice Drills are found in the back of your workbook.

1. $\dfrac{1}{7} \div \dfrac{3}{4}$

2. $\dfrac{4}{9} \div \dfrac{1}{3}$

3. $\dfrac{3}{10} \div \dfrac{5}{8}$

4. $\dfrac{6}{11} \div \dfrac{2}{5}$

5. $1\dfrac{2}{3} \div \dfrac{3}{7}$

6. $1\frac{1}{5} \div \frac{4}{9}$

7. $\frac{4}{9} \div 2\frac{1}{3}$

8. $\frac{3}{10} \div \frac{1}{8}$

9. $2\frac{3}{4} \div \frac{5}{7}$

10. $1\frac{2}{3} \div \frac{1}{4}$

11. $2\frac{3}{5} \div 5$

12. $3\frac{2}{3} \div \frac{5}{8}$

13. $1\frac{3}{5} \div \frac{3}{7}$

14. $3\frac{1}{4} \div 1\frac{2}{3}$

15. $2\frac{1}{5} \div 2\frac{1}{2}$

16. $3\frac{2}{3} \div \frac{4}{5}$

17. $1\frac{5}{6} \div 2\frac{2}{5}$

18. $5\frac{1}{2} \div 2\frac{1}{3}$

19. $6\frac{2}{3} \div 1\frac{4}{5}$

20. $3\frac{1}{4} \div 1\frac{4}{7}$

21. $1\frac{1}{3} \div \frac{1}{2}$

22. $2\frac{3}{5} \div 3$

23. $4\frac{1}{2} \div \frac{2}{5}$

24. $2\frac{4}{5} \div \frac{1}{3}$

25. $1\frac{1}{4} \div \frac{2}{7}$

26. $3\frac{2}{3} \div \frac{3}{5}$

27. $1\frac{2}{3} \div \frac{1}{4}$

28. $3\frac{2}{3} \div \frac{5}{8}$

29. $2\frac{3}{5} \div 5$

30. $2\frac{1}{4} \div \frac{2}{3}$

31. $2\frac{2}{3} \div \frac{3}{4}$

32. $4\frac{2}{5} \div 3$

33. $1\frac{3}{5} \div \frac{3}{7}$

34. $3\frac{1}{4} \div 1\frac{2}{3}$

35. $2\frac{1}{5} \div 2\frac{1}{2}$

36. $3\frac{2}{3} \div \frac{4}{5}$

37. $5\frac{1}{2} \div 2\frac{1}{3}$

38. $6\frac{2}{3} \div 1\frac{4}{5}$

39. $3\frac{1}{4} \div 1\frac{4}{7}$

40. $1\frac{5}{6} \div 2\frac{2}{5}$

REVIEW EXERCISES

Using the methods in this chapter, solve for the following problems. Return to the online course to review any content. Answers to Review Exercises are found in the back of your workbook and reduce to the lowest term.

1. $\frac{3}{5} + \frac{4}{5}$

2. $\frac{3}{10} + \frac{9}{10}$

3. $\frac{7}{9} + \frac{8}{9}$

4. $\frac{2}{3} + \frac{7}{9}$

5. $\frac{2}{3} - \frac{1}{2}$

6. $\frac{5}{6} - \frac{1}{6}$

7. $\frac{5}{6} - \frac{1}{5}$

8. $\dfrac{4}{5} - \dfrac{1}{2}$

9. $1\dfrac{1}{10} + \dfrac{3}{5}$

10. $1\dfrac{3}{8} - \dfrac{1}{2}$

11. $2\dfrac{3}{4} + 1\dfrac{2}{3}$

12. $\dfrac{3}{13} + \dfrac{4}{13}$

13. $10\dfrac{1}{6} + 7\dfrac{5}{6}$

14. $\dfrac{7}{10} + \dfrac{3}{5}$

15. $\dfrac{11}{30} + \dfrac{2}{15}$

16. $\dfrac{14}{25} + \dfrac{12}{25}$

17. $3\dfrac{1}{3} + 2\dfrac{1}{3}$

18. $\dfrac{2}{3} + \dfrac{1}{12} + 1\dfrac{1}{4}$

19. $\dfrac{2}{3} + \dfrac{7}{9} + 2\dfrac{2}{5}$

20. $11\dfrac{2}{5} + 7\dfrac{1}{2}$

21. $5\dfrac{1}{2} + 5\dfrac{1}{4}$

22. $1\dfrac{10}{11} - 1\dfrac{1}{3}$

23. $\dfrac{9}{11} - \dfrac{2}{3}$

24. $12\dfrac{1}{2} - \dfrac{3}{10}$

25. $25\dfrac{1}{3} - 20\dfrac{1}{8}$

26. $18\dfrac{3}{4} - 12\dfrac{2}{3}$

27. $20\dfrac{9}{11} - 18\dfrac{2}{3}$

28. $3\dfrac{1}{2} - 2\dfrac{2}{3}$

29. $2\dfrac{3}{4} + 1\dfrac{1}{5}$

30. $\dfrac{7}{9} \times \dfrac{4}{5}$

31. $\dfrac{1}{5} \times \dfrac{3}{7}$

32. $\dfrac{1}{9} \times \dfrac{5}{2}$

33. $2\dfrac{3}{7} \times \dfrac{1}{7}$

34. $\dfrac{4}{5} \times \dfrac{1}{20}$

35. $\dfrac{4}{5} \times 12$

36. $\dfrac{1}{4} \times 2\dfrac{5}{7}$

37. $\dfrac{9}{10} \times \dfrac{1}{3} \times \dfrac{8}{13}$

38. $1\dfrac{1}{4} \times 2\dfrac{1}{5}$

39. $2\dfrac{2}{7} \times \dfrac{11}{12}$

40. $\dfrac{1}{4} \div \dfrac{6}{7}$

41. $\dfrac{1}{3} \div 2$

42. $1\dfrac{3}{4} \div \dfrac{5}{9}$

43. $3\dfrac{3}{4} \div 1\dfrac{2}{3}$

44. $1\dfrac{7}{9} \div 1\dfrac{2}{9}$

45. $\dfrac{2}{3} \div 5$

46. $33 \div \dfrac{11}{12}$

47. $4\dfrac{3}{8} \div 3\dfrac{1}{12}$

48. $10\dfrac{6}{7} \div 7\dfrac{1}{2}$

49. $2\dfrac{1}{7} \div 2\dfrac{1}{5}$

50. $2\dfrac{1}{2} \div 2\dfrac{2}{7}$

Module **4** **Fractions**

5 | Decimals and Percents

DECIMALS

Practice Exercise 5A

Convert the following to a decimal. Return to Module 5 Screen 1.5 of the Online Course for step-by-step solutions.

1. Seven point two

2. Two and five tenths

3. 10 and 16 hundredths

4. One-hundred twenty thousandths

5. Four and seventeen thousandths

Practice Drills 5A

Answers to Practice Drills are found in the back of your workbook.
Express the following numbers to words.

1. 2.7

2. 3.54

3. 9.785

4. 15.7

5. 14.71

6. 95.312

7. 110.120

8. 45.008

9. $3,389.57

10. $4,150,070.10

Convert the following words to numbers.

11. Twelve and four tenths

12. seventy-eight and one hundred twenty-five thousandths

13. one hundred three and two hundred two thousandths

14. one thousand one hundred twenty and three hundred fifty-six thousandths

15. seventeen thousand eight hundred ninety-four and twelve hundredths

16. eighty-nine and eight thousand nine hundred fifty-two ten-thousandths

17. six hundred twelve dollars and eighty-five cents

18. two thousand four hundred dollars and forty cents

19. two hundred twenty-nine thousand three hundred forty-two dollars and ninety-five cents

20. eleven thousand five hundred ten and one thousand two hundred sixty-five ten-thousandths

Express the following numbers to words.

21. 45.6

22. 327.7

23. 13.76

24. 4.56

25. 0.8

26. 0.23

27. 3.480

28. 12.79

29. 0.153

30. 17.591

Convert the following words to numbers.

31. two and three tenths

32. six and four tenths

33. fifty-eight hundredths

34. seven hundred one thousandths

35. twelve and seventy-nine hundredths

36. forty-four and forty-six hundredths

37. forty-seven and eight-two thousandths

38. two hundred eight-two and five hundred five thousandths

39. nineteen and thirty-nine hundredths

40. three and one thousand four hundred sixteen ten-thousandths

CONVERTING BETWEEN FRACTIONS AND DECIMALS

Practice Exercise 5B

Convert the fraction or mixed number to a decimal. Return to Module 5 Screen 2.2 of the Online Course for solutions.

1. $\dfrac{1}{4}$

2. $\dfrac{3}{5}$

3. $\dfrac{17}{100}$

4. $1\dfrac{4}{5}$

5. $\dfrac{11}{2}$

Practice Drills 5B

Answers to Practice Drills are found in the back of your workbook.
Convert the fraction or mixed number to a decimal. Round to the nearest thousandths place.

1. $\dfrac{1}{100}$

2. $1\dfrac{1}{4}$

3. $\dfrac{4}{5}$

4. $4\dfrac{1}{5}$

5. $3\dfrac{4}{10}$

6. $\dfrac{11}{20}$

7. $\dfrac{9}{25}$

8. $\dfrac{55}{100}$

9. $\dfrac{7}{4}$

10. $\dfrac{6}{25}$

11. $2\dfrac{3}{5}$

12. $3\dfrac{18}{25}$

13. $4\frac{3}{50}$

14. $5\frac{1}{25}$

15. $\frac{14}{10}$

16. $3\frac{6}{25}$

17. $5\frac{3}{25}$

18. $11\frac{7}{25}$

19. $5\frac{7}{8}$

20. $4\frac{277}{1000}$

21. $\frac{32}{10}$

22. $3\frac{82}{100}$

23. $\frac{29}{50}$

24. $\frac{7}{25}$

25. $\frac{7}{11}$

26. $\frac{57}{90}$

27. $\frac{636}{1000}$

28. $\frac{63}{99}$

29. $\frac{17}{20}$

30. $1\frac{30}{100}$

31. $\frac{19}{20}$

32. $\frac{19}{20}$

33. $\frac{3}{5}$

34. $\frac{31}{40}$

50

Module **5** Decimals and Percents

35. $\dfrac{50}{41}$

36. $\dfrac{40}{17}$

37. $\dfrac{111}{200}$

38. $\dfrac{100}{97}$

39. $\dfrac{100}{63}$

40. $\dfrac{1000}{636}$

Practice Exercise 5C

Convert the following decimals to fractions. Reduce to the lowest term if needed. Return to Module 5 Screen 2.6 of the Online Course for solutions.

1. 0.5

2. 1.7

3. 98.6

4. 0.015

5. 7.04

Practice Drills 5C

Answers to Practice Drills are found in the back of your workbook.
Convert the following decimal to a fraction. Reduce to the lowest term.

1. 0.2

2. 0.375

3. 0.8

4. 1.25

5. 0.07

6. 4.2

7. 0.8511

8. 2.25

9. 0.4

10. 5.12

11. 0.06

12. 0.6

13. 4.24

14. 8.6

15. 7.625

16. 1.028

17. 9.875

18. 0.85

19. 0.125

20. 0.875

21. 0.416

22. 0.37

23. 0.90

24. 1.8

25. 3.4

26. 2.63

27. 4.39

28. 7.28

29. 0.375

30. 6.41

31. 1.372

32. 5.391

33. 8.29

34. 11.83

35. 0.864

36. 0.546

37. 1.58

38. 6.45

39. 1.43

40. 1.09

DECIMAL CALCULATIONS

Practice Exercise 5D

Add or subtract the following decimals. *Return to Module 5 Screen 3.3 of the Online Course for solutions.*

1. 2.32 + 0.14

2. 48 + 1.75

3. 0.9 + 36 + 1.25

4. 2.46 + 1.3 + 0.005

5. 14.28 + 16.24 + 97

Practice Drills 5D

Answers to Practice Drills are found in the back of your workbook.

Add or subtract the following decimals. Round to the nearest hundredths place.

1. 8.9 − 7.2

2. 9.9 + 2.1

3. 8.4 − 5.9

4. 54.7 + 9.394

5. 90 − 83.7

6. 89 + 67.9

7. 26 + 13.825

8. 76.38 − 29.75

9. 89.61 − 26.632

10. 63.59 − 27.3

11. 9.846 + 0.1938

12. 603.8 − 274.5

13. 35.71 − 28.9

14. 8.053 − 3.726

15. 6.309 − 1.954

53

16. 9.327 + 8.41

17. 0.6784 + 5 + 17.17

18. 3.256 + 27.2751 + 3.12

19. 89.61 − 26.632

20. 102.32 − 157.4 + 281.895

21. 800.54 + 90.52

22. 343.4 + 5.607

23. 94.9 − 41.871

24. 809.144 − 15.96

25. 803.309 − 133.36

26. 767.3 − 24.9

27. 489.08 − 4.2

28. 921.74 + 2.7

29. 489.08 − 4.2

30. 260.65 − 40.9

31. 384.94 + 17.348

32. 35.438 − 17.2

33. 686.4 − 199.61

34. 6.356 + 5.8

35. 75.715 + 30.5

36. 89.88 − 48.8

37. 75.715 + 30.5

38. 64.32 + 21.63

39. 875.75 + 26.64

40. 656.86 + 46.37

MULTIPLY DECIMALS

Practice Exercise 5E

Multiply the following numbers. Return to Module 5 Screen 3.6 of the Online Course for solutions.

1. 4.2×3

2. $4.75 \times .4$

3. 5.175×29.2

4. 9.708×0.17

5. 28.95×0.347

Practice Drills 5E

Answers to Practice Drills are found in the back of your workbook.

Multiply the following numbers. Round to the nearest hundredths place.

1. 2.3×4

2. 2.8×2.3

3. 0.27×7.3

4. 4.18×3

5. 21.6×15

6. 55.8×9.4

7. 0.023×80

8. 0.67×61

9. 7.91×0.19

10. 32.3×2.6

11. 61×0.46

12. 12.36×0.13

13. 68.2×8.4

14. 630×1.2

15. 0.411×0.35

16. 3.904×7.8

17. 7.514×0.58

18. 20.4×0.534

19. 117.14×212.4

20. 101.15×80.012

21. 7.8×5.1

22. -1.5×-7.1

23. 1.7×-3.1

24. 1.7×-2.1

25. 0.2×-1.6

26. -5.5×-4.87

27. -4.6×-7.2

28. -5.928×-11.6

29. $8.1 \times 8.6 \times -5.2$

30. $-4.04 \times -9 \times 3$

31. $-7.5 \times 9 \times -8.3$

32. $3.2 \times 8.7 \times -1.1$

33. 1.421×0.510

34. 7.638×9.388

35. 3.928×5

36. 9.920×1.1

37. 6.131×0.59

38. 2.396×1.171

39. 0.84×0.2268

40. 0.168×0.42

DIVIDING DECIMALS

Practice Exercise 5F

Solve for the following problems. Round to the nearest hundredths place. Return to Module 5 Screen 3.9 of the Online Course for solutions.

1. $48.6 \div 1.8$

2. $24.5 \div 0.2$

3. $1.25 \div 0.5$

56

4. $39.666 \div 0.03$

5. $29.05 \div 5.5$

Practice Drills 5F

Answers to Practice Drills are found in the back of your workbook.

Solve for the following problems. Round to the nearest hundredths place.

1. $0.05 \div 5$

2. $0.24 \div 0.3$

3. $37.6 \div 4$

4. $1.28 \div 0.4$

5. $0.54 \div 0.03$

6. $3.96 \div 0.9$

7. $38.5 \div 0.7$

8. $44.73 \div 7$

9. $61.00 \div 8$

10. $0.819 \div 0.09$

11. $9.189 \div 9$

12. $4.638 \div 0.2$

13. $37.45 \div 0.01$

14. $17.423 \div 7$

15. $588.5 \div 4$

16. $724.2 \div 0.6$

17. $84.36 \div 0.03$

18. $56.250 \div 0.9$

19. $33.672 \div 0.6$

20. $0.0568 \div 2$

21. $1.421 \div 2$

22. $0.510 \div 3$

23. $0.921 \div 2$

24. $7.638 \div 6$

25. $3.928 \div 9$

26. $9.920 \div 2$

27. $9.388 \div 8$

28. $4.334 \div 9$

29. $1.717 \div 5$

30. $0.595 \div 8$

31. $2.396 \div 4$

32. $6.131 \div 3$

33. $22.68 \div 84$

34. $57.75 \div 75$

35. $42.3 \div 94$

36. $2.28 \div 6$

37. $16.8 \div 42$

38. $0.0506 \div 0.46$

39. $0.28 \div 0.35$

40. $0.645 \div 0.86$

ROUNDING

Practice Exercise 5G

Answer the following questions. Return to Module 5 Screen 4.3 of the Online Course for solutions.

1. Round to the nearest tenth

2. Round to the nearest hundredth

3. Round to the nearest thousandth

4. Round to the nearest hundredth

5. Round to the nearest tenth

Practice Drills 5G

Answers to Practice Drills are found in the back of your workbook.
Round the following numbers to the nearest whole number.

1. 12.7

2. 71.841

3. 45.47

4. 20.36

5. 82.731

6. 12.81

7. 64.5

8. 20.35

9. 5.06

10. 16.8158

Round the following numbers to the nearest tenth.

11. 32.189

12. 66.21

13. 17.256

14. 53.93

15. 20.36

16. 0.5775

17. 0.2035

18. 0.0506

19. 0.1023

20. 0.0966

Round the following numbers to the nearest hundredth.

21. 73.414

22. 19.129

23. 87.5437

24. 52.3589

25. 21.78961

26. 49.78934

27. 94.5968

28. 7.345419

29. 21.789615

30. 53.111298

Round the following numbers to the nearest thousandth.

31. 87.5437

32. 52.3589

33. 21.78961

34. 49.78934

35. 94.5968

36. 7.345419

37. 21.789615

38. 53.111298

39. 0.5775

40. 0.0506

CONVERTING PERCENTS

Practice Exercise 5H
Convert the following numbers to either a decimal or percent. Return to Module 5 Screen 5.5 of the Online Course for solutions.

1. 0.33

2. 1.5

3. 4

4. 4%

5. 250%

Practice Drills 5H
Answers to Practice Drills are found in the back of your workbook.
Convert the following percent to a decimal.

1. 10%

2. 55%

3. 12.5%

4. 28%

5. 67%

6. 23.75%

7. 8.15%

8. 133%

9. 1.025%

10. 200.20%

Convert the following decimal to a percent.

11. 0.20

12. 0.35

13. 0.155

14. 0.125

15. 0.1575

16. 0.095

17. 0.00575

18. 0.7550

19. 1.500

20. 2.5

Convert the following percent to a decimal

21. 22.68%

22. 57.75%

23. 2.28%

24. 17.01%

25. 1.273%

26. 49.6%

27. 0.38%

28. 48.165%

29. 43.3%

30. 3.028%

Convert the following decimal to a percent.

31. 32.189

32. 66.21

33. 17.256

34. 53.93

35. 20.36

36. 0.5775

37. 0.2035

38. 0.0506

39. 0.1023

40. 0.0966

REVIEW EXERCISES

Using the methods in this chapter, solve for the following problems. Return to the online course to review any content. Answers to Review Exercises are found in the back of your workbook.

Identify which number is larger.

1. 22.12 or 21.33

2. 15.999 or 15.989

3. 0.0987 or 0.987

4. 1.001111 or 0.1110111

5. 714.8954 or 714.895401

Convert the following decimal to a fraction. Reduce to the lowest term.

6. 0.82

7. 0.250

8. 0.6155

9. 3.5

10. 1.00

Convert the following fraction to a decimal. Round to the nearest thousandths place.

11. $\dfrac{3}{10}$

12. $\dfrac{5}{8}$

13. $\dfrac{12}{10}$

14. $2\dfrac{3}{5}$

15. $5\dfrac{7}{9}$

Solve for the following problems.

16. $7.13 + 12.35$

17. $4.89 + 0.2$

18. $12 + 1.7 + 0.004$

19. $4.28 - 3.35$

20. $14.01 - 0.788$

21. $0.852 - 0.61$

22. $68.12 + 4.7$

23. $38.981 - 15.15$

24. $836 - 250.5 - 412.5$

25. $1,212.35 + 72.5 - 365.20$

26. 1.5×4

27. 7.2×1.1

28. 2.3×4.9

29. 5×0.999

30. 12.01×1.005

31. $3.8 \div 0.1$

32. $85.15 \div 0.5$

33. $38.85 \div 2.1$

34. $4.875 \div 3.25$

35. $84.3 \div 3$

Module **5** **Decimals and Percents**

Round the following numbers to the nearest tenth place.

36. 8.19

37. 5.94

38. 17.578

39. 0.8998754

40. 115.3651

Round the following numbers to the nearest hundredth place.

41. 1.011

42. 0.675

43. 0.00890

44. 6.9985

45. 15.61615

Express the following into a number.

46. two and seven tenths

47. five and seventy-five hundredths

48. seventeen and six hundred fifteen thousandths

49. twenty-five and one hundred twelve thousandths

50. one hundred and two thousand five hundred seven ten-thousandths

6 Ratios and Proportions

RATIOS

Practice Exercise 6A

Solve for the missing value (x). Return to Module 6 Screen 1.5 of the Online Course for step-by-step solutions.

1. $\dfrac{2}{3} = \dfrac{6}{x}$

2. $\dfrac{2}{x} = \dfrac{8}{100}$

3. $10 : x = 5 : 8$

4. $10 : 4 = 10 : x$

5. It takes 150 minutes to walk 10 miles. How long would it take to walk 35 miles?

Practice Drills 6A

Answers to Practice Drills are found in the back of your workbook.
Convert the following to ratios.

1. $\dfrac{1}{2}$

2. $\dfrac{4}{5}$

3. $1\dfrac{1}{2}$

4. $1\dfrac{9}{10}$

5. $\dfrac{15}{5}$

6. 75%

7. 90%

8. 5

9. $\dfrac{1}{100}$

10. 100%

11. $\dfrac{10}{1}$

12. 10%

13. $\dfrac{15}{100}$

14. There are 8 slices in a pizza. You have eaten 4 slices.

15. Twenty minutes in an hour

16. A day in a week

17. A month in a year

18. A family has 5 children. Three of the children are girls.

19. A patient takes 2 aspirins from a bottle with 60 tablets

20. A venue has capacity for 500 people. Its capacity is at 20%.

21. 20%

22. 85%

23. 99%

24. 110%

25. 201%

26. $\dfrac{10}{1}$

27. $\dfrac{15}{3}$

28. $\dfrac{1}{15}$

29. $\dfrac{1}{100}$

30. $\dfrac{2}{12}$

31. An auditorium has 100 seats and 80% of them are occupied. What is the ratio of occupancy?

32. A shoe of a pair of shoes

33. An egg in a carton of eggs

34. Thumbs on two hands

35. A dime out of one dollar

36. A math club has 25 members, of which 11 are males and the rest are females. What is the ratio of males to all club members?

37. A group of preschoolers has 8 boys and 24 girls. What is the ratio of girls to all children?

38. A pattern has 4 blue triangles to every 12 yellow triangles. What is the ratio of blue triangles to all triangles?

39. A club has 21 members, of which 13 are males and the rest are females. What is the ratio of females to all club members?

40. A group of preschoolers has 63 boys and 27 girls. What is the ratio of boys to all children?

PROPORTIONS

Practice Exercise 6B

Convert the fraction or mixed number to a decimal. Return to Module 6 Screen 2.4 of the Online Course for step-by-step solutions.

1. $\dfrac{1}{4}$

2. $\dfrac{3}{5}$

3. $\dfrac{17}{100}$

4. $1\dfrac{4}{5}$

5. $\dfrac{11}{2}$

Practice Drills 6B

Answers to Practice Drills are found in the back of your workbook.
Solve for χ. Round to the nearest hundredths place.

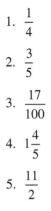

1. $\dfrac{1}{2} = \dfrac{2}{\chi}$

2. $\dfrac{\chi}{26} = \dfrac{3}{13}$

3. $\dfrac{1}{4} = \dfrac{10}{\chi}$

4. $\dfrac{2}{3} = \dfrac{\chi}{18}$

5. $\dfrac{\chi}{8} = \dfrac{8}{64}$

6. $\dfrac{3}{\chi} = \dfrac{27}{45}$

7. $\dfrac{2}{21} = \dfrac{\chi}{84}$

8. $\dfrac{\chi}{72} = \dfrac{15}{27}$

9. $\dfrac{\chi}{32} = \dfrac{20}{8}$

10. $\dfrac{3}{7} = \dfrac{6}{\chi}$

11. $\dfrac{11}{22} = \dfrac{\chi}{110}$

12. $\dfrac{2}{\chi} = \dfrac{12}{18}$

13. $\dfrac{50}{20} = \dfrac{5}{\chi}$

14. $\dfrac{5}{\chi} = \dfrac{20}{50}$

15. $\dfrac{\chi}{6} = \dfrac{5}{7}$

16. $\dfrac{7}{\chi} = \dfrac{11}{12}$

17. $\dfrac{10}{21} = \dfrac{\chi}{5}$

18. $\dfrac{3}{7} = \dfrac{\chi}{37}$

19. $\dfrac{2}{9} = \dfrac{\chi}{19}$

20. $\dfrac{12}{33} = \dfrac{61}{\chi}$

21. $\dfrac{20}{6} = \dfrac{\chi}{9}$

22. $\dfrac{10}{\chi} = \dfrac{6}{8}$

23. $\dfrac{7}{9} = \dfrac{\chi}{6}$

24. $\dfrac{7}{6} = \dfrac{2}{\chi}$

25. $\dfrac{8}{\chi} = \dfrac{4}{8}$

26. $\dfrac{6}{\chi} = \dfrac{8}{2}$

27. $\dfrac{\chi}{9} = \dfrac{7}{3}$

28. $\dfrac{2}{\chi} = \dfrac{12}{18}$

29. $\dfrac{50}{20} = \dfrac{5}{\chi}$

30. $\dfrac{16}{6} = \dfrac{\chi}{3}$

31. $\dfrac{45}{27} = \dfrac{\chi}{3}$

32. $\dfrac{9}{3} = \dfrac{\chi - 10}{8}$

33. $\dfrac{\chi - 1}{5} = \dfrac{8}{2}$

68

34. $\dfrac{8}{5} = \dfrac{3}{\chi - 8}$

35. $\dfrac{2}{9} = \dfrac{10}{\chi - 4}$

36. $\dfrac{9}{\chi + 2} = \dfrac{3}{9}$

37. $\dfrac{\chi + 10}{7} = \dfrac{1}{4}$

38. $\dfrac{\chi - 5}{15} = \dfrac{4}{5}$

39. $\dfrac{16}{6} = \dfrac{3\chi}{9}$

40. $\dfrac{20}{8} = \dfrac{4\chi}{32}$

REVIEW EXERCISES

Using the methods in this chapter, solve for the following problems. Return to the online course to review any content. Answers to Review Exercises are found in the back of your workbook.
Round to the nearest hundredths place.
Convert the following to ratios.

1. $\dfrac{2}{3}$

2. $\dfrac{3}{10}$

3. $\dfrac{3}{2}$

4. $\dfrac{10}{100}$

5. $3\dfrac{1}{3}$

6. 75%

7. 4%

8. 0.65

9. 1.15

10. 250%

11. A quarter in a dollar

12. 5 minutes in an hour

Convert the following ratios to fractions or mixed numbers. Remember to reduce to the lowest term.

13. 5:6

14. 2:12

15. 10:15

16. 7:3

17. 9:5

18. 5:75

19. 38:12

Convert the following ratios to a percent.

20. 2:3

21. 1:4

22. 2:9

23. 20:1

24. 15:2

25. 1:50

26. 5:2

27. 25:100

28. 250:100

29. 3:1000

Write the following in a proportion.

30. $\dfrac{3}{4} = \dfrac{9}{12}$

31. $\dfrac{5}{10} = \dfrac{500}{1000}$

32. $\dfrac{5}{6} = \dfrac{10}{12}$

33. $\dfrac{3}{8} = \dfrac{15}{40}$

34. $\dfrac{10}{2} = \dfrac{50}{10}$

Determine if the following proportions are valid or not valid.

35. $1:2 = 3:6$

36. $20:50 = 400:100$

37. $\dfrac{2}{10} = \dfrac{10}{25}$

38. $\dfrac{5}{8} = \dfrac{40}{72}$

39. $5 : 25 = 10 : 250$

Solve for the missing value (x).

40. $10 : x = 5 : 8$

41. $10 : 4 = 20 : x$

42. $x : 24 = 5 : 30$

43. $\dfrac{200}{100} = \dfrac{x}{500}$

44. $\dfrac{3x}{4} = \dfrac{48}{8}$

45. $\dfrac{2x}{20} = \dfrac{12}{50}$

46. $\dfrac{15x}{8} = \dfrac{360}{120}$

47. A recipe calls for 3 cups of flour to bake a cake. How much flour would you need to bake two cakes?

48. A patient is prescribed 2 pills a day. How many pills will the patient take for 2 weeks?

49. A loaf of bread costs $2.50. How much bread can you buy with $30?

50. One gallon of gas costs $3. Your car can hold 15 gallons. How much does it cost to fill the tank of gas?

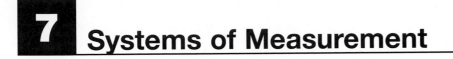

7 Systems of Measurement

STANDARD HOUSEHOLD SYSTEM

Practice Exercise 7A

Solve for the following questions. Return to Module 7 Screen 1.8 of the Online Course for step-by-step solutions.

1. How many ounces are in a cup?

2. How many pints are in 2 quarts?

3. How many tablespoons are in 8 ounces?

4. How many cups are in a quart?

5. How many pints are in 3 quarts?

Practice Drills 7A

Answers to Practice Drills are found in the back of your workbook.
Convert the following measurements.

1. 16 gal = _____ pt.

2. 15 qt = _____ pt.

3. 16 qt = _____ gal.

4. 7 gal = _____ c

5. 8 qt = _____ pt

6. 16 c = _____ qt

7. 16 oz = _____ pt

8. 32 pt = _____ qt

9. 48 c = _____ qt

10. 128 oz = _____ c

11. 656 oz. = _____ lbs.

12. 27 lbs. = _____ oz.

13. 992 oz. = _____ lbs.

14. 36 in = _____ ft

15. 540 in = _____ ft

16. 52 ft = _____ in

17. 18 ft = _____ yd

18. 1.7 mi = _____ yd

19. 1,750 yd = _____ mi

20. 0.45 mi = _____ ft

21. 35.4 lbs. = _____ oz

22. 35 qt = _____ gal

23. 77.1 lbs. = _____ oz

24. 62.37 lbs. = _____ oz

25. 868 oz = _____ lbs.

26. 664 yd = _____ mi

27. 450 yd = _____ mi

28. 0.69 mi = _____ yd

29. 17,656 ft = _____ mi

30. 3,573 yd = _____ mi

31. 5,527 ft = _____ mi

32. 543 ft = _____ mi

33. 6,298 yd = _____ mi

34. 8 mi = _____ ft

35. 42.3 mi = _____ yd

36. 2 oz = _____ lb

37. 4 c = _____ oz

38. 27 ft = _____ yd

39. 1,777 ft = _____ mi

40. 25 gal = _____ qt

Using the methods in this chapter, solve for the following problems. Return to the online course to review any content. Answers to Review Exercises are found in the back of your workbook.
For Questions #1-5, write the amount and unit abbreviations for the following:

1. fourteen pounds

2. fifty-two and five tenths ounces

3. eight-hundred thirteen grains

4. sixteen and one-half tablespoons

5. two-hundred fifteen gallons

6. Convert 1 tablespoon to teaspoon

7. Convert 32 ounces to pounds

8. Convert 2 cups to ounces

9. Convert 1 pound to ounce

10. Convert 1 pint to ounce

11. Convert $3\frac{1}{4}$ cups to ounces.

12. Convert 12 ounces to tablespoons.

13. Convert 1 gallon to cups.

14. Convert $2\frac{1}{3}$ tablespoons to drops.

15. Convert 1 cup to teaspoons.

16. Convert 1 pint to tablespoons

17. Convert 2 cups to ounces

18. Convert 5 ounces to grains

19. Convert 5 tablespoons to drams

20. Convert 2 pounds to grains

21. 1 gal = _____ c

22. 8 c = _____ gal

23. 6 gal = _____ qt

24. 64 c = _____ qt

25. 32 oz = _____ qt

26. 3 gal = _____ qt

27. 6 mi = _____ ft

28. 5 mi = _____ yd

29. 52 ft = _____ in

30. 65 ft = _____ in

31. 240 in = _____ ft

32. 444 in = _____ ft

33. 12 yds = _____ ft

34. 45 yds = _____ ft

35. 35 ft = _____ yd

36. 102 ft = _____ yd

37. 216 ft = _____ yd

38. 108 in = _____ yd

39. 65 ft = _____ in

40. 504 in = _____ yds

41. 6 yds = _____ ft

42. 672 in = _____ ft

43. 24 yds = _____ in

44. 432 oz = _____ lbs.

45. 38 lbs. = _____ oz

46. 640 oz = _____ lbs.

47. 52 lbs. = _____ oz

48. 48 oz = _____ lbs.

49. 96 oz = _____ lbs.

50. 51 lbs. = _____ oz.

8 | The Metric System

STRUCTURE OF THE METRIC SYSTEM

Practice Exercise 8A

Translate the following to either a word or abbreviation. Return to Module 8 Screen 1.3 of the Online Course for answers.

1. km

2. mcg

3. cm

4. milliliter

5. decimeter

Answers to Practice Drills are found in the back of your workbook.
This should be placed after Practice Drills 8A.

Practice Drills 8A

Write the correct abbreviation for each metric unit.

1. meter

2. gram

3. liter

4. kilometer

5. milligram

6. centimeter

7. hectogram

8. millimeter

9. microliter

10. decigram

Determine if the following units are used to measure *liquid*, *weight*, or *length*.

11. grams

12. liters

13. mg

14. milliliters

15. meter

16. kg

17. mL

18. km

19. mcg

20. cm

Write the correct metric unit for each abbreviation.

21. L

22. cm

23. km

24. mg

25. m

26. kg

27. mL

28. mcg

29. m

30. dg

31. g

32. cL

33. kL

34. dm

35. dL

36. dag

37. dal

38. cg

39. hL

40. dam

Practice Exercise 8B
Write the indicated amounts using numbers and abbreviations. Return to Module 8 Screen 1.6 of the Online Course for step-by-step solutions.

1. Eighty-two centimeters

2. Twenty-two micrograms

3. Seven and one-half milliliters

4. Three-hundredths of a gram

5. Seven-tenths of a meter

Practice Drills 8B
Answers to Practice Drills are found in the back of your workbook.
Write the number and abbreviations for the following measurements.

1. Five liters

2. Fifteen kilometers

3. One hundred fifteen centimeters

4. Fifty-two centigrams

5. Thirty milliliters

6. One thousand grams

7. One thousandth milligram

8. Fifty thousand micrograms

9. Two and four tenths grams

10. Forty-nine and nine-tenths of a kilogram

Identify which of the following number is larger or equal.

11. 5 kiloliters or 5 liters

12. 5 microliters or 5 milliliters

13. 100 centimeters or 100 millimeters

14. 52 centigrams or 52 milligrams

15. 30 milliliters or 30 kilometers

16. 15 dm or 15 mm

17. 49.9 hl or 49.9 kl

18. 1,000 gr or 100,000 mg

19. 0.001 mg or 10 mcg

20. 50,000,000 mcg or 5 kg

Define the following abbreviations.

21. 1.31 kL

22. 2.64 hm

23. 100 mg

24. 3.53 hL

25. 908 dal

26. 0.27 mm

27. 125 cg

28. 1,546 cm

29. 10 dag

30. 18 cL

Identify which of the following number is larger or equal.

31. 1.31 kL or 13.1 L

32. 2.64 hm or 264 cm

33. 100 mg or 0.1 kg

34. 3.53 hL or 3.53 kL

35. 908 dL or 9,008 L

36. 0.27 mm or 0.27 cm

37. 125 cg or 1.25 g

38. 1,546 cm or 15.46 m

39. 10 dag or 100 hg

40. 18 cL or 0.0018 kL

Practice Exercise 8C

Convert the following. Return to Module 8 Screen 1.9 of the Online Course for step-by-step solutions.

1. Convert 4 kilograms to gram

2. Convert 50 centimeters to milliliters

3. Convert 0.75 gram to milligram

4. Convert 14 centimeters to meter

5. Convert 0.4 kilogram to milligram

Practice Drills 8C

Answers to Practice Drills are found in the back of your workbook.
Convert the following.

1. 2 L = _____ mL

2. 1 cl = _____ L

3. 1,000 L = _____ kL

4. 46 mL = _____ L

5. 110 g = _____ kg

6. 53 cm = _____ mm

7. 0.085 g = _____ mg

8. 355 mL = _____ L

9. 160 cm = _____ mm

10. 109 g = _____ kg

11. 950 mm = _____ dm

12. 2 kg = _____ g

13. 3.4 hm = _____ m

14. 1 dekaliter = _____ liters

15. 14 km = _____ m

16. 250 m = _____ km

17. 120 mg = _____ g

18. 455 mL = _____ L

19. 63 cm = _____ mm

20. 43 mg = _____ kg

21. 1.31 km = _____ m

22. 2.64 hm = _____ dm

23. 100 mg = _____ g

24. 3.53 hL = _____ kL

25. 908 daL = _____ L

26. 0.27 mm = _____ hm

27. 125 cg = _____ g

28. 1,546 cm = _____ km

29. 10 dag = _____ mg

30. 18 cL = _____ mL

31. 220 cg = _____ kg

32. 3.527 mL = _____ hL

33. 15.43 km = _____ m

34. 1.25 g = _____ hg

35. 109.36 dg = _____ mg

36. 39.37 dam = _____ m

37. 0.39 dag = _____kg

38. 0.04 kg = _____ dm

39. 3,861 hL = _____ L

40. 155 kg = _____ dam

CONVERTING BETWEEN MEASUREMENT SYSTEMS

Practice Exercise 8D

Convert the following. Return to Module 8 Screen 2.3 of the Online Course for step-by-step solutions.

1. Convert 4 ounces to milliliters.

2. Convert 66 pounds to kilograms.

3. Convert 720 milliliters to pints.

82

4. Convert 4 cups to milliliters.

5. Convert 2 teaspoons to milliliters.

Practice Drills 8D
Answers to Practice Drills are found in the back of your workbook.
Convert the following.

1. 3 kg = _____ lb.

2. 22 lb. = _____ kg

3. 15 lb. = _____ kg

4. 10 lb. = _____ kg

5. 9 kg = _____ lb.

6. 16 lb. = _____ oz.

7. 70 kg = _____ lb.

8. 640 oz. = _____ lb.

9. 1 ft = _____ cm

10. 5 ft = _____ cm

11. 9 ft = _____ cm

12. 3 yd = _____ cm

13. 1 yd = _____ cm

14. 4 m = _____ ft

15. 6 ft = _____ m

16. 20 ft = _____ m

17. 5 cm = _____ in

18. 1 pt = _____ mL

19. 475 mL = _____ c

20. 475 mL = _____ oz.

21. 45 in = _____ cm

22. 25.3 m = _____ ft

23. 2.3 mi = _____ km

24. 14 in = _____ cm

25. 125 lbs. = _____ kg

26. 20 gal = _____ L

27. 16 in = _____ cm

28. 345 lbs. = _____ kg

29. 56 g = _____ oz

30. 453 km = _____ mi

31. 1,200 mL = _____ oz

32. 40 m = _____ ft

33. 4 gal -= _____ L

34. 12 oz = _____ mL

35. 50 kg = _____ lbs.

36. 19 cm = _____ in

37. 200 kg = _____ lbs.

38. 60 miles = _____ km

39. 355 mL = _____ oz

40. 1 lb. = _____ g

REVIEW EXERCISES

Using the methods in this chapter, solve for the following problems. Return to the online course to review any content. Answers to Review Exercises are found in the back of your workbook.

Translate the following to either a number or words.

1. forty-two and nine tenth grams

2. six-hundred twenty-five kilometers

3. seventeen hundredth milligram

4. 7.5 cm

5. 102.15 mL

Identify which of the following number is larger or equal.

6. 42 L or 420 mL

7. 10 cm or 1,000 mm

8. 15.5 mg or 1 kg

9. 1 qt or 1 L

10. 1 m or 1 yd

11. 3.4 m or 309 cm

12. 1.95 km or 1,564 m

13. 43 mg or 5 g

14. 3.6 m or 3.6 cm

15. 1.5 m or 127 cm

16. 2,800 mm or 28 cm

17. 1,240 m or 1.3 km

18. 14 mm or 1.8 cm

19. 12 km or 6 miles

20. Convert 7.5 mg to mcg

Convert the following measurements.

21. Convert 0.750 mL to L

22. Convert 500 g to mg

23. Convert 3.75 g to mg

24. Convert 0.0055 L to mL

25. Convert 1.2 mm to cm

26. Convert 600 mL to L

27. Convert 1 cup to mL

28. Convert 2 Tb. to mL

29. Convert 15 mL to tsp.

30. Convert 360 mL to oz.

31. Convert 12 lbs. to kg

32. Convert 0.6 L to oz.

33. 88 kg = _____ lb.

34. 54 kg = _____ lb.

35. 29 kg = _____ lb.

36. 42 kg = _____ lb.

37. 32 lb. = _____ oz.

38. 11 tsp. = _____ oz.

39. 12.5 in. = _____ cm

40. 76 cm = _____ in

41. 6.4 m = _____ yd

42. 20 ft = _____ m

43. 15 m = _____ ft

44. 10 m = _____ yd

45. 260 in = _____ yd

46. 150 cm = _____ ft

A pharmacy is preparing a prescription for azithromycin, an antibiotic, for a child. The antibiotic is an oral dose and is prescribed as 30 milliliters.

47. How many tablespoons should be taken?

48. How many teaspoons should be taken?

A medical assistant is taking the measurements of an infant for a growth chart. The infant is 0.445 m. and 7.3 kg. What is the baby's weight in inches and pounds?

49. _____ in.

50. _____ lbs.

9 Temperature and Time

TEMPERATURE

Practice Exercise 9A
Convert the following to either °C or °F. Return to Module 9 Screen 1.6 of the Online Course for answers.

1. Convert 102 °F to °C

2. Convert 125 °F to °C

3. Convert 41 °C to °F

4. Convert 42.6 °C to °F

5. Convert 67 °C to °F

Practice Drills 9A
Answers to Practice Drills are found in the back of your workbook.
Convert the following temperatures to either °F or °C.

1. 0 °C = _____ °F

2. 100 °C = _____ °F

3. 58 °F = _____ °C

4. 15 °F = _____ °C

5. 33 °F = _____ °C

6. 85 °F = _____ °C

7. 14 °C = _____ °F

8. 20 °C = _____ °F

9. 9 °C = _____ °F

10. 36 °F = _____ °C

11. 56 °F = _____ °C

12. 66 °C = _____ °F

13. 33 °C = _____ °F

14. 88 °F = _____ °C

15. 4 °C = _____ °F

16. 95 °F = _____ °C

17. 87 °C = _____ °F

18. The patient's temperature is 100.5 °F. What is her temperature in C?

19. The boiling point of water is 212 °F. What is it in C?

20. What is the freezing point of water in C?

21. 25 °C = _____ °F

22. 45 °C = _____ °F

23. 0 °C = _____ °F

24. 20 °C = _____ °F

25. 90 °C = _____ °F

26. 40.3 °C = _____ °F

27. 65 °C = _____ °F

28. 102 °F = _____ °C

29. 37 °F = _____ °C

30. 200 °F = _____ °C

31. 175 °F = _____ °C

32. 185 °F = _____ °C

33. 158 °F = _____ °C

34. 68 °F = _____ °C

35. 194 °F = _____ °C

36. 67 °C = _____ °F

37. 78 °F = _____ °C

38. 48 °C = _____ °F

39. The temperature in Phoenix was recorded as 80.6 °F. What is the temperature in degree Celsius on that day?

40. In the month of June, the hottest temperature in Houston was recorded as 42.4 °C. Convert it into degree Fahrenheit.

Practice Exercise 9B

Convert the times in the table. *Return to Module 9 Screen 2.8 of the Online Course for answers.*

	12-Hour Time	24-Hour Time
1.	2:35 a.m.	
2.	3:14 p.m.	
3.		3:25
4.		00:11
5.		15:25

Practice Drills 9B

Answers to Practice Drills are found in the back of your workbook.
Convert the following to either 12-hour clock (include a.m. or p.m.) or 24-hour clock.

1. 6:00 a.m. = _____

2. 2:45 a.m. = _____

3. 2:45 p.m. = _____

4. 11:30 a.m. = _____

5. 6:20 = _____

6. 13:10 = _____

7. 17:30 = _____

8. 14:36 = _____

9. 2:12 = _____

10. 12:15 p.m. = _____

11. 11:45 a.m. = _____

12. 11:12 p.m. = _____

13. 20:36 = _____

14. 1:25 p.m. = _____

15. 10:50 = _____

16. 16:41 = _____

17. 5:02 p.m. = _____

18. 1:56 a.m. = _____

19. 21:12 = _____

20. 3:47 = _____

21. Based on the clock in Figure 9.1, what time is it for a 12-hour clock?

22. Based on the clock in Figure 9.1, what time is it for a 24-hour clock?

    Morning: _____

    Nighttime: _____

23. Based on the clock in Figure 9.2, what time is it for a 12-hour clock?

24. Based on the clock in Figure 9.2, what time is it for a 24-hour clock?

    Morning: _____

    Nighttime: _____

25. Based on the clock in Figure 9.3, what time is it for a 12-hour clock?

26. Based on the clock in Figure 9.3, what time is it for a 24-hour clock?

    Morning: _____

    Nighttime: _____

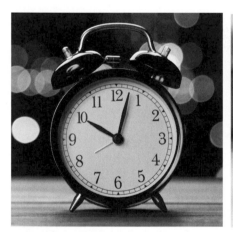

Figure 9.1 © iStock.com/
GeorgeDolgikh

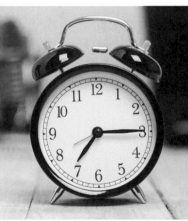

Figure 9.2 © iStock.com/picture

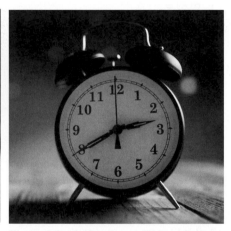

Figure 9.3 © iStock.com/BrianAJackson

Convert the following to a 24-hour clock.

27. 11:15 p.m.

28. 8:37 a.m.

29. 9:25 p.m.

30. 7:45 a.m.

31. 5:53 a.m.

32. 1:30 p.m.

Convert the following to a 12-hour clock (include a.m. or p.m.).

33. 10:15

34. 7:38

35. 11:05

36. 20:45

37. 13:00

38. 3:37

39. 22:30

40. 6:36

Practice Exercise 9C
Solve for the following questions.

1. How many minutes are in 1 week?

2. How many seconds are in 1 day?

3. How many months are in 7 years?

4. How many weeks are in a decade?

5. How many days are in 4 months?

Practice Drills 9C
Answers to Practice Drills are found in the back of your workbook.
Convert the following units.

1. 2 hours = _____ minutes

2. 10 hours = _____ minutes

3. 360 minutes = _____ hours

4. 540 minutes = _____ hours

5. 210 minutes = _____ hours

6. 10.25 hours = _____ minutes

7. 10 minutes = _____ seconds

8. 16 minutes = _____ seconds

9. 180 seconds = _____ minutes

10. 300 seconds = _____ minutes

11. 900 seconds = _____ minutes

12. 2 days = _____ hours

13. 96 hours = _____ days

14. 384 hours = _____ days

15. 13 days = _____ hours

16. $\frac{1}{2}$ hour = _____ seconds

17. 3 years = _____ months

18. 3 years = _____ weeks

19. 3 years = _____ days

20. 3 years = _____ seconds

21. 8 minutes = _____ seconds

22. 5 days = _____ hours

23. 10 days = _____ hours

24. 9 hours = _____ minutes

25. 7 days = _____ hours

26. 240 minutes = _____ hours

27. 216 hours = _____ days

28. 360 seconds = _____ minutes

29. 168 hours = _____ days

30. 300 seconds = _____ minutes

31. 24 hours = _____ days

32. 480 minutes = _____ hours

33. 3 days = _____ hours

34. 2 weeks = _____ days

35. 120 seconds = _____ minutes

36. 6 hours = _____ minutes

37. 5 days = _____ hours

38. 10 hours = _____ minutes

39. 13 hours 45 minutes = _____ minutes

40. 5 weeks 4 days = _____ days

REVIEW EXERCISES

Using the methods in this chapter, solve for the following problems. Return to the online course to review any content. Answers to Review Exercises are found in the back of your workbook.

1. Convert 78.3 °F to °C.

2. Convert 18.2 °C to °F

3. Convert 25.8 °C to °F

4. Convert 72 °F to °C

5. Convert 400 °F to °C

6. Convert 25 °C to °F

7. Convert 95 °C to °F

8. Convert 122 °F to °C

9. The freezing temperature at:
   _____ °C
   _____ °F

10. The boiling temperature at:
    _____ °C
    _____ °F

11. Convert 4:17 a.m. to 24-hour time

12. Convert 4:50 p.m. to 24-hour time

13. Convert 11:10 p.m. to 24-hour time

14. Convert 12:59 a.m. to 24-hour time

15. Convert 0029 to 12-hour time

16. Convert 0912 to 12-hour time

17. Convert 2055 to 12-hour time

18. 11:45 = _____

19. 4:13 a.m. = _____

20. 19:05 = _____

Use the clock below to answer Questions #21-23.

What time is it?

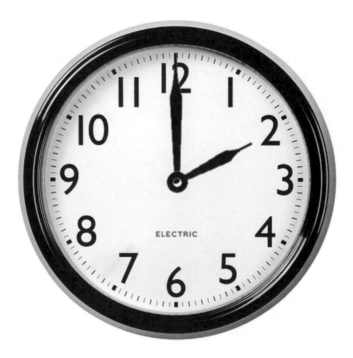

21. 12-hour clock: _____

22. Using the 24-hour clock, what time is it in the morning?

23. Using the 24-hour clock, what time is it in the evening?

Use the clock below to answer Questions #24-25.

What time is it?

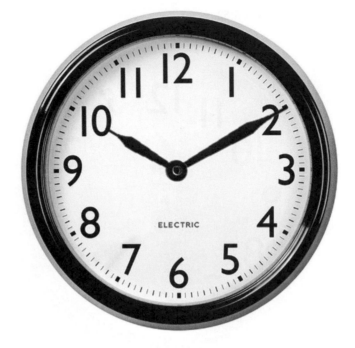

24. 12-hour clock: _____

25. Using the 24-hour clock, what time is it in the morning?

Using the 24-hour clock, what time is it in the evening?

What time is it?

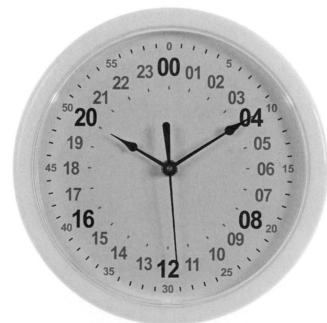

26. 24-hour clock: _____

12-hour clock: _____

27. On the clock, draw the hands to represent 8:52.

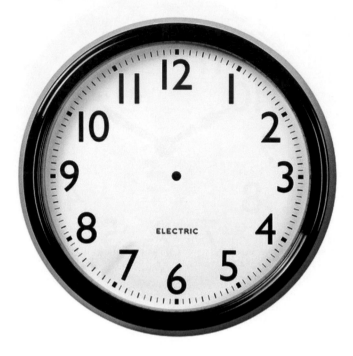

© iStock.com/RTimages

28. On the 24-hour clock, draw 6:30 p.m.

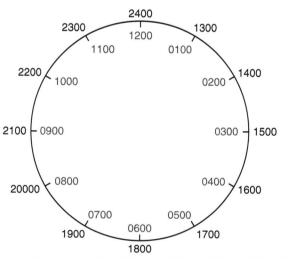

Modified from Potter PA, Perry AG: *Fundamentals of nursing*, ed 10, St. Louis, 2021, Elsevier.

Convert the following units.

29. 4 hours = _____ minutes

30. 6 hours = _____ day

31. $\frac{3}{4}$ day = _____ hours

32. $\frac{3}{4}$ day = _____ seconds

33. $\frac{1}{2}$ a year = _____ weeks

34. $\frac{1}{2}$ a year = _____ days

35. 7 min = _____ sec

36. 1.5 min = _____ sec

37. 5 hours = _____ min

38. 600 min = _____ hours

39. 305 min = ___ h ___ min

40. 110 min = ___ h ___ min

41. 700 min = ___ h ___ min

42. 5 h 20 min = _____ min

43. 2 h 10 min = _____ min

44. 6 h 45 min = _____ min

45. 6 weeks = _____ days

46. 98 days = _____ weeks

47. 50 days = ___ weeks ___ days

48. 87 days = ___ weeks ___ days

49. 210 days = ___ weeks ___ days

50. 5 months 5 days = _____ days

10 Prescriptions and Drug Calculations

MEDICATION ORDERS, PRESCRIPTIONS, AND LABELS

Practice Exercise 10A

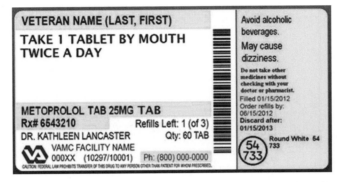

From U.S. Department of Veterans Affairs Website. A New and Improved VA Prescription Label. Available at https://www.va.gov/health/newsfeatures/2015/january/a-new-and-improved-va-prescription-label.asp. Accessed January 23, 2022.

Use the drug label to answer the following questions. Return to Module 10 Screen 1.15 of the Online Course for answers.

1. What is the name of the medication?

2. What is the dosage?

3. What is the route of administration?

4. How often should the patient take the medication?

5. How many tablets are dispensed?

6. How many refills is this patient allowed after this prescription?

Practice Drills 10A
Answers to Practice Drills are found in the back of your workbook.
For Questions #1-5, determine if the answer is brand or generic name.

1. The medication's name assigned by the drug manufacturer

2. Every medication must have one

3. The medication name must be capitalized

4. The medication name is usually first and not in parentheses

5. The medication's name is assigned by the United States Adopted Names Council

Use the prescription in Fig. 10.1 to answer Questions #6-10.

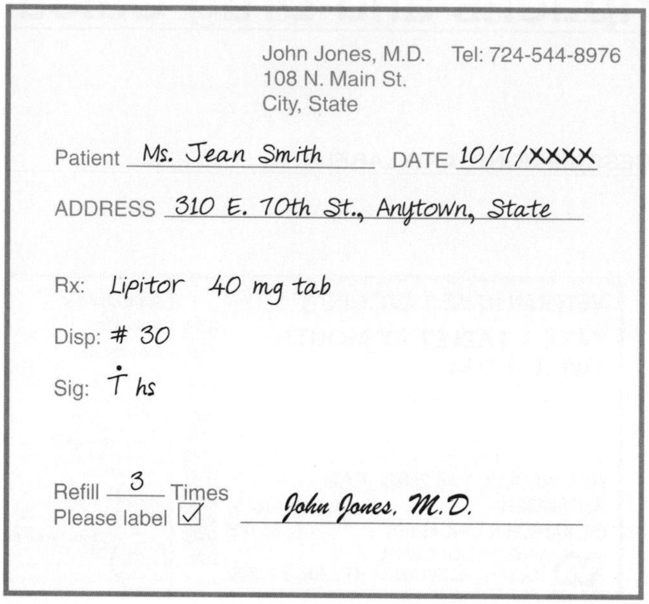

John Jones, M.D. Tel: 724-544-8976
108 N. Main St.
City, State

Patient Ms. Jean Smith DATE 10/7/XXXX
ADDRESS 310 E. 70th St., Anytown, State

Rx: Lipitor 40 mg tab
Disp: # 30
Sig: $\dot{T}$ hs

Refill 3 Times
Please label ☑ John Jones, M.D.

Figure 10.1. From Proctor DB, et al.: *Kinn's the clinical medical assistant: an applied learning approach*, ed 13, St. Louis, 2017, Elsevier.

6. What is the name of the drug?
7. What is the prescribed dosage?
8. What is the amount dispensed?
9. What is the route of administration for this drug?
10. How many refills are allowed in this prescription?

Use the prescription in Fig. 10.2 to answer Questions #11-20.

Caroline A. Fann, M.D.
198 Dean's Way
Four Corners, N.C. 26362
(199) 377-7157

DEA#

Name Eve R. Bluehook Age 47
Address 877 Rapp Bypass Date 4-28-01
Rx (Please print)
enalapril 5 mg tabs
disp: #30
Sig: one daily
Always label
Refill 5 Times
Product selection permitted M.D. Caraline A ferr M.D. Dispense as written

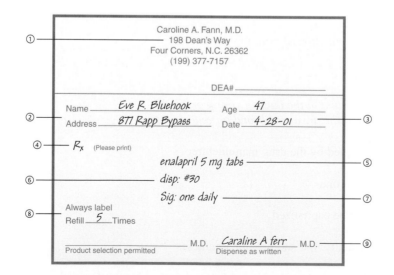

Figure 10.2

List which number identifies the information.

11. Superscription

12. Inscription

13. Patient's name

14. Signatura (Sig)

15. What is the name of the medication?

16. What is the recommended dosage?

17. What is the route of administration?

18. What is the frequency of the medication?

19. What is the amount dispensed?

20. How many refills are permitted?

Use the prescription in Fig. 10.3 to answer Questions #21-26.

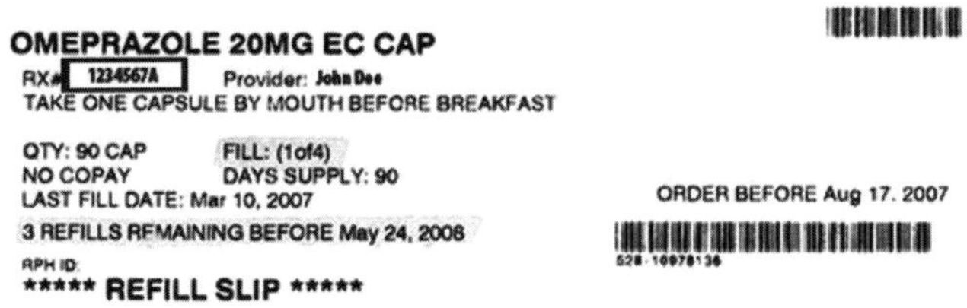

OMEPRAZOLE 20MG EC CAP
RX# 1234567A   Provider: John Doe
TAKE ONE CAPSULE BY MOUTH BEFORE BREAKFAST

QTY: 90 CAP   FILL: (1of4)
NO COPAY   DAYS SUPPLY: 90
LAST FILL DATE: Mar 10, 2007
3 REFILLS REMAINING BEFORE May 24, 2008
RPH ID:
***** REFILL SLIP *****

ORDER BEFORE Aug 17. 2007

528-10970136

Figure 10.3

21. What is the name of the medication?

22. What is the recommended dosage?

23. What is the route of administration?

24. What is the frequency of the medication?

25. What is the amount dispensed?

26. How many refills are permitted?

Use the prescription in Fig. 10.4 to answer Questions #27-34.

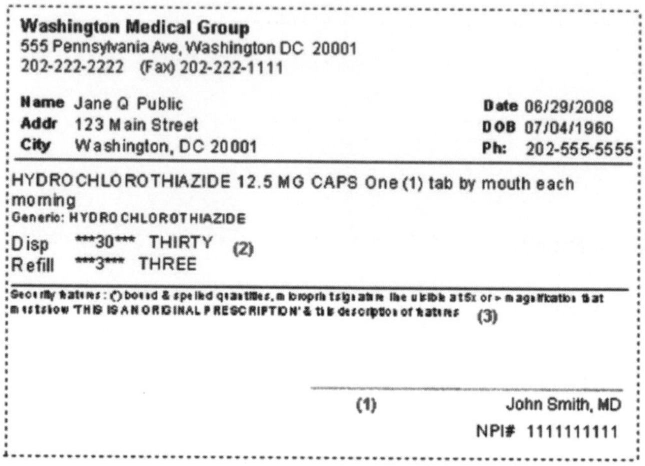

Washington Medical Group
555 Pennsylvania Ave, Washington DC 20001
202-222-2222 (Fax) 202-222-1111

Name Jane Q Public   Date 06/29/2008
Addr 123 Main Street   DOB 07/04/1960
City   Washington, DC 20001   Ph: 202-555-5555

HYDROCHLOROTHIAZIDE 12.5 MG CAPS One (1) tab by mouth each
morning
Generic: HYDROCHLOROTHIAZIDE

Disp   ***30*** THIRTY   (2)
Refill   ***3***   THREE

Security features: () bordsd & spelled quantities, m broprh tsigi atsre the usible at5x or > magsrfkatios that m sstslow THIS IS AN ORDINAL PRESCRIPTION & tit descrsptios of satsnf   (3)

_____
                        (1)   John Smith, MD
                                                     NPI# 1111111111

Figure 10.4. From North Dakota Department of Human Services: Medicaid Tamper-Resistant Prescription Requirements. Available at https://www.nd.gov/dhs/services/medicalserv/medicaid/docs/pharmacy/trpp-pharmacist-edu-and-faqs.pdf. Accessed January 24, 2022.

27. What is the name of the medication?

28. What is the recommended dosage?

29. What is the route of administration?

30. What is the frequency of the medication?

31. What is the amount dispensed?

32. How many refills are permitted?

33. What is the patient's name?

34. What is the prescriber's name?

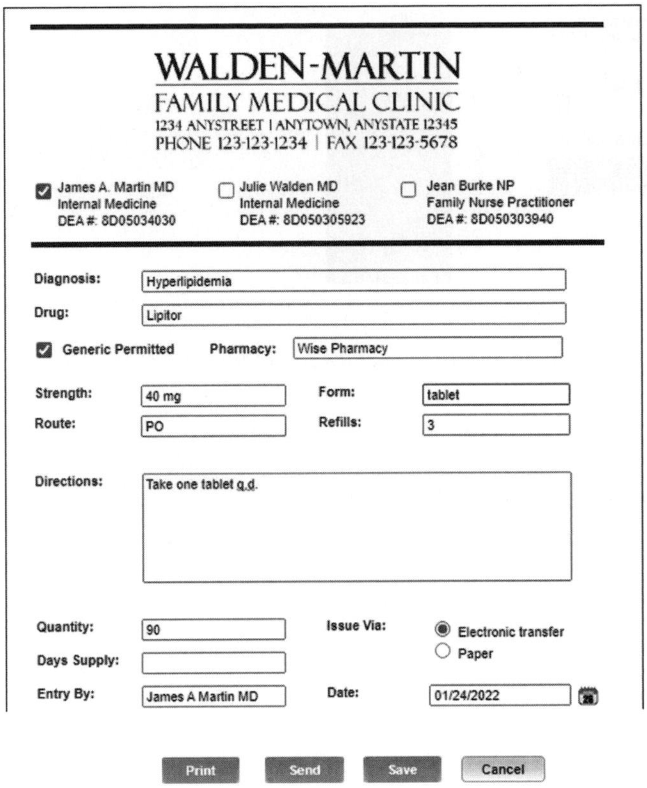

WALDEN-MARTIN
FAMILY MEDICAL CLINIC
1234 ANYSTREET | ANYTOWN, ANYSTATE 12345
PHONE 123-123-1234 | FAX 123-123-5678

☑ James A. Martin MD   ☐ Julie Walden MD   ☐ Jean Burke NP
Internal Medicine   Internal Medicine   Family Nurse Practitioner
DEA #: 8D05034030   DEA #: 8D050305923   DEA #: 8D050303940

Diagnosis: Hyperlipidemia

Drug: Lipitor

☑ Generic Permitted   Pharmacy: Wise Pharmacy

Strength: 40 mg   Form: tablet
Route: PO   Refills: 3

Directions: Take one tablet q.d.

Quantity: 90   Issue Via: ● Electronic transfer
Days Supply: ○ Paper
Entry By: James A Martin MD   Date: 01/24/2022

Print   Send   Save   Cancel

Figure 10.5.   From SimChart © 2022, Elsevier, Inc.

Use the prescription in Fig. 10.5 to answer Questions #35-40.

35. What is the name of the medication?

36. What is the recommended dosage?

37. What is the route of administration?

38. What is the frequency of the medication?

39. What is the amount dispensed?

40. How many refills are permitted?

Practice Exercise 10B

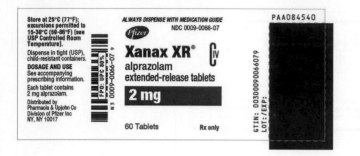

Use the drug label to answer the following questions. Return to Module 10 Screen 1.17 of the Online Course for answers.

1. The drug's generic name is _____.

2. The drug's brand name is _____.

3. What is the dosage?

4. What is the quantity?

5. What is the drug form?

Practice Drills 10B
Answers to Practice Drills are found in the back of your workbook.

NEIGHBORHOOD PHARMACY
193 MAIN ST   HOUSTON, PA 11111   (555) 123-4567

RX # 6001103   RB   DR. D. ASH
SMITH, JOHN   00/00/0000
193 MAIN ST   HOUSTON, PA 11111
TAKE TWO TABLETS BY MOUTH 2 TIMES A DAY

120 METFORMIN HCL 500 MG TABL

NO REFILLS
NDC# 1234567890   ORIG: 08/27/XX

Figure 10.6

Figure 10.6 Prescription Question s #1-10
Use the drug label in Fig. 10.6 to answer Questions #1-10.

1. What is the name of the patient?

2. What is the name of the prescriber?

3. What is the name of the prescribed medication?

104

4. What is the dosage of the medication in each tablet?

5. What is the route of administration?

6. What is the abbreviation for the route of administration?

7. What is the frequency of the prescribed medication?

8. What is the abbreviation?

9. How many tablets are dispensed with this prescription?

10. How many refills are allowed in this prescription?

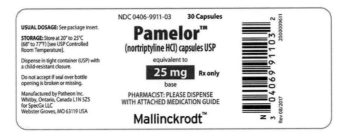

Figure 10.7

Use the drug label in Fig. 10.7 to answer Questions #11-20.

11. What is the generic name of the medication?

12. What is the brand name of the medication?

13. What is the dosage?

14. What is the drug form of this medication?

15. What is the route of administration?

16. How many capsules are dispensed?

17. If the patient takes this medication "as needed," what is the abbreviation for this frequency?

18. If the patient takes this medication three times a day, what is the abbreviation for this frequency?

19. The patient is instructed to take the medication QD. How many capsules will he need each month?

20. The patient is instructed to take the medication BID. How many refills will he need in one month?

Use the drug label in Fig 10.8 to answer Questions #21-30.

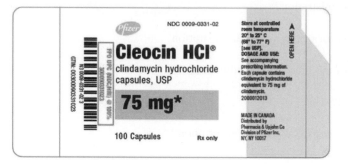

Figure 10.8

21. What is the generic name of the medication?

22. What is the brand name of the medication?

23. What is the dosage of the drug?

24. What is the drug form of this medication?

25. What is the route of administration?

26. How many capsules are dispensed?

27. If the patient takes this medication every 4 hours, what is the abbreviation for this frequency?

28. The patient is instructed to take the medication every 4 hours. How many days will the dosage on hand supply?

29. If the patient is prescribed to take this medication every 4 hours, how many refills will he need for 1 month?

Use the drug label in Fig. 10.9 to answer Questions #30-34.

30. What is the brand name of the medication?

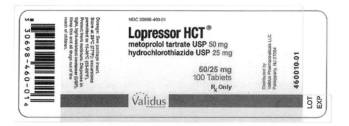

Figure 10.9

31. What is the dosage of the metoprolol?

32. How many tablets are dispensed?

33. If the patient is prescribed this drug BID, how many days will this supply?

34. If the patient is prescribed this drug BID, what is the patient's daily dosage?

Use the drug label in Fig 10.10 to answer Questions #35-40.

35. What is the generic name of the medication?

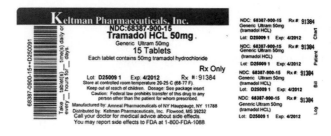

Figure 10.10

36. What is the dosage of the drug?

37. How many tablets are dispensed?

38. What is the expiration date of the drug?

39. If the patient is prescribed this drug q8h, how many days will this supply?

40. If the patient is prescribed this drug q8h, how many refills will the patient need for 1 month?

DOSAGE CALCULATIONS

Practice Exercise 10C

Solve for the following questions. Return to Module 10 Screen 2.3 of the Online Course for answers.

1. The medication order is for 30 mg PO QD of a medication. The dosage of the supply on hand is 10 mg per tablets. How many tablets should the patient take each day?

2. The medication order is for 1,500 mg PO QD of a medication. The dosage of the supply on hand is 500 mg per tablets. How many tablets should the patient take each day?

3. The medication order is for 0.25 g. PO QD of a medication. The dosage on hand is 50 mg in 2 milliliters. How much should the patient take each day?

4. The physician prescribes 20 mg per milliliters of a liquid cough syrup. The label on the cough syrup shows the dosage to be 10 mg per milliliters. How many milliliters should the patient take each day?

5. You only have a teaspoon. How much medication in Question #4 should you take in teaspoon?

Practice Drills 10C

Answers to Practice Drills are found in the back of your workbook.

Solve for the following questions.

Phenobarbital, an anticonvulsant drug, is prescribed for 30 mg PO QD. The drug on hand is 30 mg tablets.

1. What is the desired dose?

2. What is the strength or supply on hand?

3. What is the medication's unit of measurement or quantity of unit?

4. How many tablets should the patient take?

A patient is prescribed Procardia (nifedipine) 20 mg PO daily. What is on hand is 10 mg capsules.

5. What is the desired dose?

6. What is the strength or supply on hand?

7. What is the medication's unit of measurement or quantity of unit?

8. How many tablets should the patient take?

Use the drug label in Fig 10.11 to answer Questions #9-14.

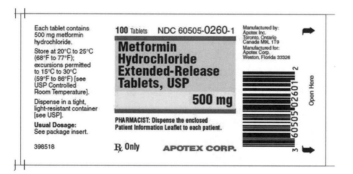

Figure 10.11

A patient is prescribed metformin 1,000 mg PO BID.

9. What is the desired dose?

10. What is the strength or supply on hand?

11. What is the medication's unit of measurement or quantity of unit?

12. How many tablets should the patient take at one time?

13. How many tablets should the patient take every day?

14. What is the patient's daily dosage?

The prescribed dosage is 500 mg q6h. The dosage on hand is 250 mg per tablet.

15. How many tablets should the patient take?

16. What is the patient's daily dosage?

17. How many tablets should the patient take per day?

The patient is prescribed nitroglycerin 800 mcg tablets sublingual PRN. The dosage on hand is 0.4 mg tablets.

18. What is the desired dosage in mg?

19. How many tablets should the patient take?

20. How should the patient take this tablet?

21. A drug is ordered at 30 mg. On hand is 10 mg tablets. How much should be administered?

22. A drug is ordered at 1 mg. On hand is 5 mg/mL. How much should be administered?

23. A drug is ordered at 1,500 mg. On hand is 500 mg tablets. How much should be administered?

24. A drug is ordered at 15 mg. On hand is 7.5 mg tablets. How much should be administered?

25. A drug is ordered at 10 mg. On hand is 20 mg/mL. How much should be administered?

26. A drug is ordered at 0.25 g. On hand is 50 mg/2 mL. How much should be administered?

27. A drug is ordered at 1.5 mg. On hand is 3 mg/mL. How much should be administered?

28. A drug is ordered at 0.1 g. On hand is 25 mg/2 mL. How much should be administered?

29. A drug is ordered at 0.15 g. On hand is 25 mg tablets. How much should be administered?

30. A drug is ordered at 10 mg. On hand is 2.5 mg tablets. How much should be administered?

31. A drug is ordered at 1 g. On hand is 50 mg/2 mL. How much should be administered?

32. A drug is ordered at 0.5 g. On hand is 200 mg tablets. How much should be administered?

33. A drug is ordered at 0.15 g. On hand is 300 mg tablets. How much should be administered?

34. A drug is ordered at 0.06 g. On hand is 15 mg tablets. How much should be administered?

35. A drug is ordered at 1.5 g. On hand is 125 mg/2 mL. How much should be administered?

36. A drug is ordered at 1.5 g. On hand is 1,000 mg tablets. How much should be administered?

37. A drug is ordered at 1.5 g. On hand is 750 mg tablets. How much should be administered?

38. Zoloft (sertraline) is ordered at 200 mg. On hand is 50 mg tablets. How much should be administered?

39. Docusate is ordered at 300 mg. On hand is 150 mg/15 mL. How much should be administered?

40. Cozaar (losartan) is ordered at 100 mg. On hand is 25 mg tablets. How much should be administered?

109

Using the methods in this chapter, solve for the following problems. Return to the online course to review any content. Answers to Review Exercises are found in the back of your workbook.

Define the following routes of administration.

1. oral

2. transdermal

3. buccal

4. sublingual

5. parenteral

Define the following abbreviations or convert to an abbreviation.

6. QD

7. TID

8. PRN

9. twice a day

10. q4h

Use the drug label to answer the Questions #11-18.

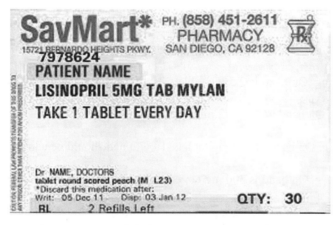

From California Board of Pharmacy. The Script. March 2012. Available at https://www.pharmacy.ca.gov/publications/12_mar_script.pdf. Accessed January 23, 2022.

11.   What is the name of the drug?

12. What is the prescribed or desired dosage?

13. What is the drug form?

14. What is the route of administration?

15. What is the quantity dispensed?

16. How many refills were provided?

17. What is the medication abbreviation for "once every day"?

18. What is the drug dosage the patient will be taking every day?

Use the drug label to answer Questions #19-27.

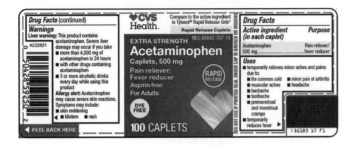

19. Acetaminophen is the _____ name of the drug.

20. What is the quantity?

21. What is the drug form?

22. What is the drug dosage in each caplet?

For a healthy average adult, the general recommended maximum daily dose of acetaminophen is 4,000 mg.

23. What is the maximum number of acetaminophens can a health adult take each day?

24. Based on the dosage formula, what is the D?

25. Based on the dosage formula, what is the H?

26. Based on the dosage formula, what is the Q?

27. What is the maximum number of caplets an adult should take each day?

Use the following drug label to answer Questions #28-35.

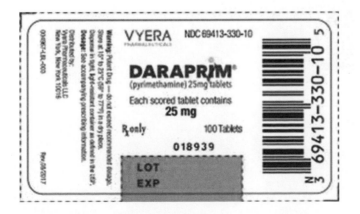

The medication order is for the patient to take 25 mg Daraprim PO TID.

28. Daraprim is the _____ name of this drug.

29. How many mg of the drug is in each pill?

30. How many times a day should the patient take the drug?

31. What is the desired dose?

32. What is the strength or supply on hand?

33. What is the drug's dosage unit?

34. How many tablets should the patient take each day?

35. What is the patient's total dosage per day?

Use the drug label below for Questions #36-37.

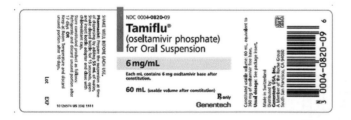

The physician prescribes 500 mg cephalexin PO BID.

36. What is the patient's daily drug dosage?

37. How many capsules should the pharmacy provide for a month's supply of the medication?

Use the drug label below for Questions #38-39.

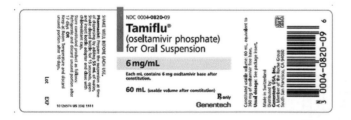

The patient is prescribed Tamiflu 75 mg BID for 5 days.

38. How much should the patient take based on the prescription?

39. How much Tamiflu will the patient need patient need based on the prescription?

Use the drug label below for Questions #40-42.

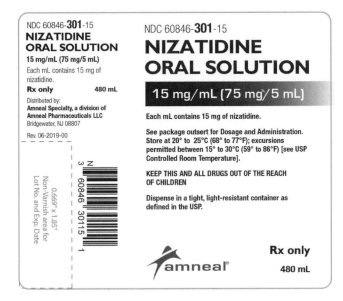

A patient is prescribed nizatidine for gastric ulcers. The prescription is for 75 mg PO BID.

40. How much should the patient take?

41. What is the daily desired dose?

42. How much drug is in the container?

Solve for the following questions.

43. Erythromycin is ordered at 0.5 g. On hand is 500 mg tablets. How much should be administered?

44. Penicillin is ordered at 0.25 g. On hand is 500 mg tablets. How much should be administered?

45. Biaxin (clarithromycin) is ordered at 1 g PO daily. On hand is 500 mg tablets. How much should be administered?

46. Synthroid (levothyroxine) is ordered at 0.05 mg. On hand is 50 mcg tablets. How much should be administered?

47. Norvir (ritonaviro) is ordered at 200 mg PO. On hand is 80 mg/mL. How much should be administered?

48. Clarithromycin is ordered at 7.5 mL PO q4h. On hand is 125 mg/5 mL. What is the dosage administered?

49. Levothroid is ordered at 0.112 mg. On hand is 112 mcg tablets. How much should be administered?

50. Risperdal (risperidone) is ordered at 750 mcg. On hand is 0.5 mg tablets. How much should be administered?

LIQUID DRUG FORMS

Practice Exercise 11A

Use the drug label to answer the following questions. Return to Module 11 Screen 1.7 of the Online Course for answers.

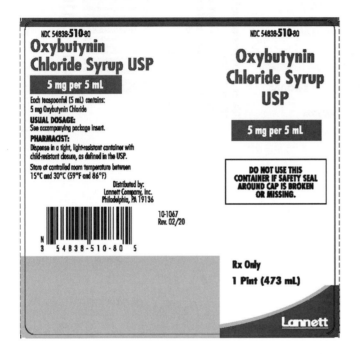

1. Is oxybutynin chloride the brand name or generic name of this drug?

2. What is the quantity on hand of this drug?

3. What is the dosage of this drug?

4. The medication order is 10 mg. How much should the patient take?

5. The medication order is 2.5 mg. How much should the patient take?

Practice Drill 11A

Answers to Practice Drills are found in the back of your workbook.
Use the drug label in Fig. 11.1 to answer Questions #1-9.

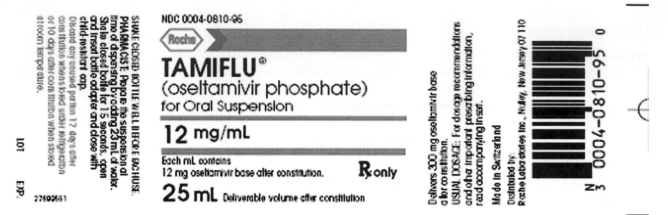

Figure 11.1

1. What is the generic name of the drug?

2. What is the brand name of this drug?

3. What is the route of administration?

4. What is the quantity on hand of this drug?

5. What is the dosage of this drug?

6. The adult dosage is 75 mg PO QD. How much should the patient take?

7. Based on the quantity on hand, how many dosages can the adult patient take?

8. The pediatric dosage for a child 1-12 years of age is 30 mg PO QD. How much should the patient take?

9. Based on the quantity on hand, how many dosages can the pediatric patient take?

Use the drug label in Fig. 11.2 to answer Questions #10-13.

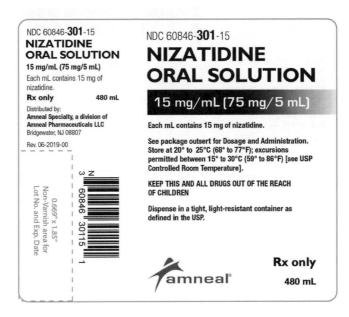

Figure 11.2

10. How much of the drug is in 1 mL?

11. The recommended dosage of nizatidine for gastroesophageal reflux diseases (GERD) is 150mg PO q12hr. How much should the patient take each time?

12. How often should the patient take this medication each day?

13. What is the patient's daily dosage of medication?

Use the drug label in Fig. 11.3 to answer Questions #14-17.

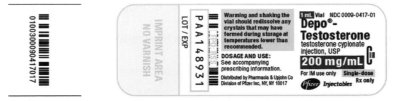

Figure 11.3

Depo-Testosterone is used as a replacement therapy for males with deficient or absence of testosterone. The recommended dosage is 50-400mg administered every two to four weeks.

14. The patient is being prescribed an intramuscular (IM) injection for 50 mg. How much should be injected?

15. If the patient is prescribed 50 mg every two weeks, how many dosages does the vial contain?

16. If the physician decides to increase the dosage to 350 mg, how much should be administered?

Module **11 Weight-Based Dosage Calculations**

17. If the patient is prescribed 400 mg, how many dosages does the vial contain?

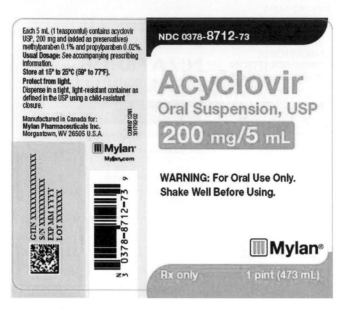

Figure 11.4

Use the drug label in Fig. 11.4 to answer Questions #18-20.

18. Acyclovir is being prescribed to at 800 mg PO QID. How much should the patient take each dosage?

19. What is the patient's daily drug dosage each day?

20. How many total dosages is on hand?

21. A patient is prescribed 500 mg of a Neurontin (gabapentin) oral solution. The drug on hand is 250 mg/5 mL How much should be administered?

22. A patient is prescribed ephedrine sulfate 12.5 mg SC. The drug on hand is 25 mg/mL How much should be administered?

23. A patient is prescribed diazepam 2 mg IM. The drug on hand is 5 mg/mL How much should be administered?

24. A patient is prescribed amitriptyline 25 mg IM. The drug on hand is 10 mg/mL How much should be administered?

25. A patient is prescribed Loxitane (loxapine) 30 mg IM. The drug on hand is 50 mg/mL How much should be administered?

26. A patient is prescribed atropine 0.6 mg IM. The drug on hand is 0.8 mg/mL How much should be administered?

27. A patient is prescribed Dilaudid 0.5 mg IM. The drug on hand is 2 mg/mL How much should be administered?

28. A patient is prescribed Zantac (ranitidine) 35 mg IM. The drug on hand is 35 mg/mL How much should be administered?

29. A patient is prescribed 0.25 g of a medication. The drug on hand is 50 mg/2 mL How much should be administered?

30. A patient is prescribed 20 mg of a medication. The drug on hand is 10 mg/5 mL How much should be administered?

31. A patient is prescribed 50 mg of a medication. The drug on hand is 12.5 mg/5 mL How much should be administered?

32. A patient is prescribed 60 mg of cough syrup. The label on the cough syrup shows 100 mg/5 mL. How much should be administered?

33. A patient is prescribed 0.25 g of a medication. The drug on hand is 50 mg/2 mL How much should be administered?

34. A patient is prescribed 1.5 mg of a medication. The drug on hand is 3 mg/mL How much should be administered?

35. A patient is prescribed 0.1 g of a medication. The drug on hand is 25 mg/2 mL How much should be administered?

36. A patient is prescribed 1 g of a medication. The drug on hand is 50 mg/2 mL How much should be administered?

37. A patient is prescribed 1.5 g of a medication. The drug on hand is 125 mg/2 mL How much should be administered?

38. A patient is prescribed 125 mg of a medication. The drug on hand is 100 mg/4 mL How much should be administered?

39. A patient is prescribed 75 mg of a medication. The drug on hand is 25 mg/2 mL How much should be administered?

40. A patient is prescribed colchicine 0.5 mg of a medication. The drug on hand is 500 mcg/mL How much should be administered?

WEIGHT-BASED DOSAGES AND SPECIAL UNIT DOSAGES

Practice Exercise 11B

Solve for the following questions. Return to Module 11 Screen 2.3 of the Online Course for answers.

1. A medication order is for 2mg/kg of a drug is required in a single dose. The patient weights 36 kg. How many milligrams should you administer to the patient?

2. The physician order is 12 mg/kg of a drug. The patient weights 115 lbs. The drug is supplied as 100 mg/2 mL. How much should you administer to the patient?

3. The nurse practitioner writes a medication order for 15 mL of acetaminophen oral suspension PO QID. How much of the drug will the patient consume a day? (Use the drug label in Fig. 11.5.)

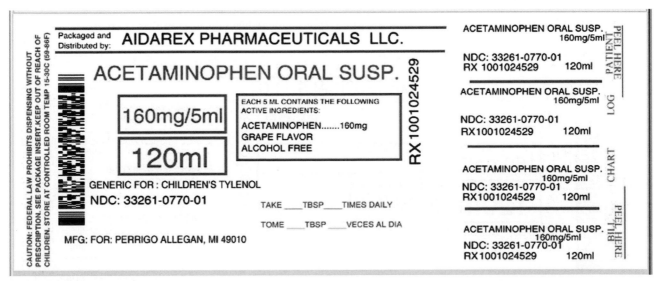

Figure 11.5

4. Amoxicillin is prescribed at 35 mg/kg for 24 hours in 3 divided doses. The patient's weight is 12 kg. The drug on hand is 125 mg in 5 ml suspension. How many milliliters (mL) will you administer in a single dose?

119

5. The physician assistant prescribes 50 mg/kg of cephalexin to a child. The child is 85 lbs. How much should the child drink? (Use the drug label in Fig. 11.6)

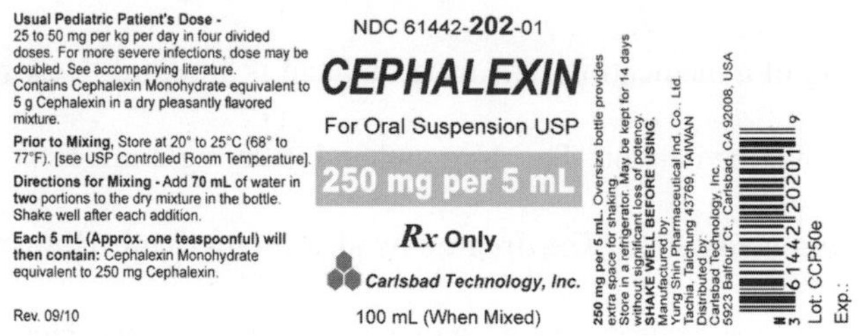

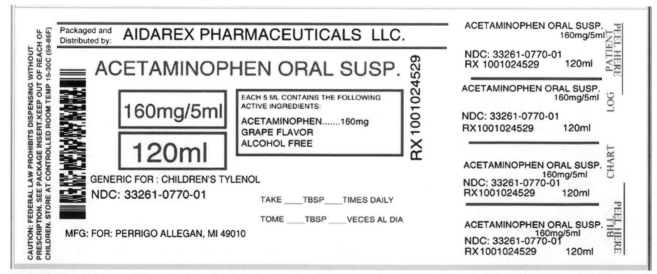

Figure 11.6

Practice Drill 11B

Solve for the following problems. Round to the nearest tenth place. Answers to Practice Drills are found in the back of your workbook.

Amoxicillin is prescribed at 35 mg/kg. The patient's weight is 12 kg.

1. How much amoxicillin should the patient receive?

2. The drug on hand is 125 mg in 5 ml suspension. How many milliliters (mL) will you administer?

The physician order is 12 mg/kg of a drug. The patient weights 115 lbs. The drug is supplied as 100 mg/2 mL.

3. What is the patient's weight in kilograms?

4. How much drug should the patient receive?

5. How much drug should be administered?

Use drug label in Fig. 11.7 for Questions #6-11.
The nurse practitioner writes a medication order for 15 mL of acetaminophen oral suspension PO QID.

Figure 11.7

6. A child receives 10 mL of acetaminophen. How much drug did the child receive?

7. A child is prescribed 400 mg of acetaminophen. How much should be administered?

8. An infant weights 15 lbs. How much is this in kilograms?

9. The pediatrician prescribes the infant 10 mg/kg acetaminophen PO q6h. How much of the drug should the infant receive per dose?

10. How much acetaminophen should be administered to the infant?

11. Per the guidelines based on the infant's age, the daily dosage of acetaminophen should not exceed 2.6 g in 24 hours. Per the prescription, what is this infant's daily dosage? Does this exceed the recommended daily dosage?

Use the label in Fig 11.8 for Questions #12-14.

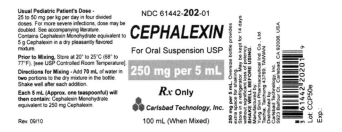

Figure 11.8

12. The child is 85 lbs. How much does the child weight in kilograms?

13. The physician assistant prescribes 50 mg/kg of cephalexin to the child. What is the dosage prescribed?

14. How much of the drug should be administered to the child?

Use the drug label in Fig 11.4 to answer Questions #15-19.
The recommended dose of oral acyclovir for a child with chickenpox is 10-20 mg/kg four times a day for 5 to 7 days.

15. The child weights 35 lbs. What is the child's weight in kilograms?

16. A child with chickenpox is prescribed 20 mg/kg. How much acyclovir is in each dosage?

17. How much acyclovir should be administered to the child per dose?

18. What is the child's daily dosage of acyclovir?

19. How much acyclovir is in the bottle?

Solve for the following questions.

20. A medication order is for 2mg/kg of a drug is required in a single dose. The patient weights 36 kg. How many milligrams should you administer to the patient?

Module **11** **Weight-Based Dosage Calculations**

21. A patient is prescribed 15 mg/kg of a drug. The patient weights 8 lbs. How much should be administered?

22. A patient is prescribed 100 mg/kg of a drug. The patient weights 24 lbs. How much should be administered?

23. A patient is prescribed 0.25 mg/kg of a drug. The patient weights 18 lbs. How much should be administered?

24. A patient is prescribed ampicillin 30 mg/kg of a drug. The patient weights 22 lbs. How much should be administered?

25. A patient is prescribed 5 mg/kg of a drug. The patient weights 14 lbs. How much should be administered?

26. A patient is prescribed 1.5 mg/kg of a drug. The patient weights 78 lbs. How much should be administered?

27. A patient is prescribed 2 mg/kg of a drug. The patient weights 42 lbs. How much should be administered?

28. A patient is prescribed 2.5 mg/kg of a drug. The patient weights 35 lbs. How much should be administered?

29. A patient is prescribed Valium (diazepam) 7.5 mg IM. The drug on hand is 0.2 mg/kg. The patient weights 175 lbs. How much should be administered?

30. A patient is prescribed 0.1 mg/kg of a drug. The patient weights 17 lbs. How much should be administered?

31. A patient is prescribed 2 mg/kg of a drug. The patient weights 108 lbs. How much should be administered?

32. A patient is prescribed 12 mg/kg of a drug. The patient weights 16.5 lbs. How much should be administered?

33. A patient is prescribed 0.5 mg/kg of a drug. The patient weights 32.5 lbs. How much should be administered?

34. A patient is prescribed 0.25 mcg/kg of a drug. The patient weights 19 lbs. How much should be administered?

35. A patient is prescribed Ativan (lorazepam) 800 mcg IM. The drug on hand is 0.05 mg/kg. The patient weights 85 lbs. How much should be administered?

36. A patient is prescribed 0.2 mg/kg of a drug. The patient weights 125 lbs. How much should be administered?

37. A patient is prescribed 0.5 mg/kg. The patient weights 165 lbs. How much should be administered?

38. A patient is prescribed 16 mg/kg of a drug. The patient weights 24lbs. 4 oz. How much should be administered?

39. A patient is prescribed 15 mg/kg of a drug. The patient weights 8 lbs. How much should be administered?

40. A patient is prescribed 0.25 mcg/kg of a drug. The patient weights 6 lbs. 8 oz. How much should be administered?

Practice Exercise 11C

Use the drug label in Fig 11.9 to answer the following questions. Return to Module 11 Screen 2.7 of the Online Course for answers.

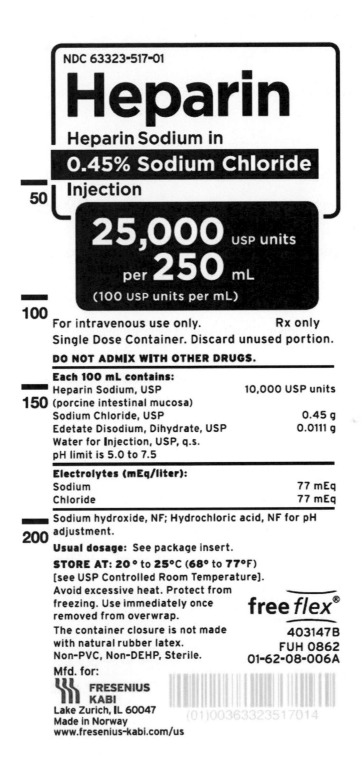

NDC 63323-517-01

Heparin

Heparin Sodium in
0.45% Sodium Chloride
Injection

50

25,000 USP units
per **250** mL
(100 USP units per mL)

100

For intravenous use only.   Rx only
Single Dose Container. Discard unused portion.

DO NOT ADMIX WITH OTHER DRUGS.

Each 100 mL contains:
Heparin Sodium, USP   10,000 USP units
(porcine intestinal mucosa)

150
Sodium Chloride, USP   0.45 g
Edetate Disodium, Dihydrate, USP   0.0111 g
Water for Injection, USP, q.s.
pH limit is 5.0 to 7.5

Electrolytes (mEq/liter):
Sodium   77 mEq
Chloride   77 mEq

Sodium hydroxide, NF; Hydrochloric acid, NF for pH
200 adjustment.

Usual dosage: See package insert.

STORE AT: 20° to 25°C (68° to 77°F)
[see USP Controlled Room Temperature].
Avoid excessive heat. Protect from
freezing. Use immediately once   free*flex*®
removed from overwrap.
                                           403147B
The container closure is not made   FUH 0862
with natural rubber latex.   01-62-08-006A
Non-PVC, Non-DEHP, Sterile.

Mfd. for:

FRESENIUS
KABI
Lake Zurich, IL 60047   (01)00363323517014
Made in Norway
www.fresenius-kabi.com/us

Figure 11.9

1. Based on the drug label, how can heparin be administered?

2. How much heparin is in 1 mL?

3. How much heparin is contained in the vial?

4. The medication order is for heparin 15,000 IU SC BID. What is the dosage of heparin the patient will be administered every day?

5. A medication order is for the patient to receive heparin 8,000 IU SC every 8 hours. How many mL of heparin does he receive daily?

Practice Drill 11C

Solve for the following problems. Answers to Practice Drills are found in the back of your workbook.

1. The patient is prescribed heparin 10,000 units. The heparin on hand is 5,000 units/mL. How many mL should be administered?

2. A patient is prescribed heparin of 4,000 units. The heparin on hand is 1,000 units/mL. How many mL should be administered?

3. Heparin is prescribed at 60 units/kg. The patient is 80 kg. How many units should the patient receive?

4. A patient is to receive a heparin drip of 18 units/kg. The patient weights 75 kg. How many units should the patient receive?

5. The patient is prescribed 18 units/kg. The patient's weight is 167 lbs. How much heparin should be administered?

6. A medication order is for heparin at 40 mL/hr. The heparin on hand is 40,000 U in 1,000 mL. How many units are in 40 mL?

A patient is prescribed heparin of 14 units/kg. The heparin on hand is 1,000 units/mL. The patient weights 203 lbs.

7. How many units should the patient receive?

8. How many mL should be administered to the patient?

Heparin is dosed at 70 units/kg for a 130-lb female. Heparin is available at 1,000 units/mL.

9. How many units should the patient receive?

10. How many mL should be administered?

Use the drug label in Fig 11.10 to answer Questions #11-15.

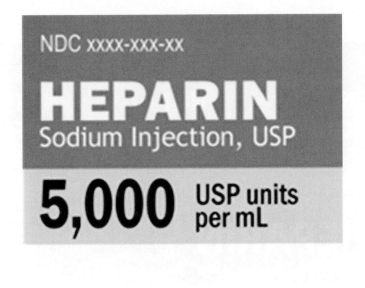

Figure 11.10

11. Based on the drug label, how can heparin be administered?

12. How much heparin is in 1 mL?

13. How much heparin is contained in the vial?

14. The medication order is for heparin 15,000 IU SC BID. What is the dosage of heparin the patient will be administered every day?

15. A patient is prescribed heparin at 24 mL/hr. The heparin on hand is 12,500 units/250 mL. How many units should the patient receive?

An order to start heparin at 60 units/kg. The heparin supplied is 25,000 units/250 mL. The patient weights 189 lbs.

16. How many units should the patient receive?

17. How many mL should the patient receive?

Module **11** **Weight-Based Dosage Calculations**

Use the drug label in Fig 11.11 to answer Questions #18-20.

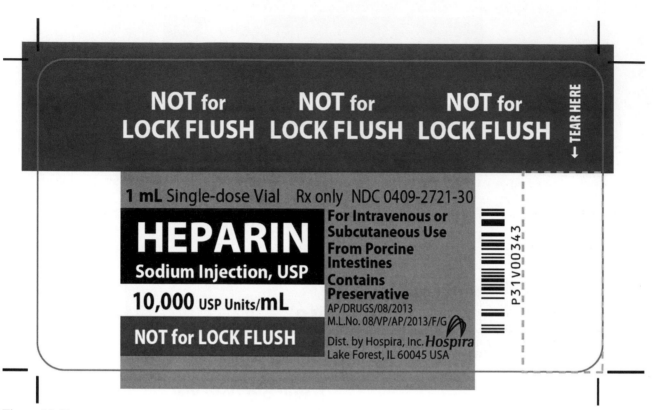

Figure 11.11

18. A patient is prescribed a heparin bolus of 15,000 units. How much should be administered?

19. The physician prescribes heparin at 75 units/kg. The patient weight 155 lb. How much should be administered?

20. How many mL should the patient receive?

Solve for the following problems.

21. A patient is prescribed heparin 2,500 units SC. The drug on hand is 5,000 units/mL. How much should be administered?

22. A patient is prescribed heparin 5,000 units. The drug on hand is 10,000 units/mL. How much should be administered?

23. A patient is prescribed penicillin G 100,000 units. The drug on hand is 1,000,000 units/5mL. How much should be administered?

24. A patient is prescribed heparin 15,000 units. The drug on hand is 1,000 units/mL. How much should be administered?

25. A patient is prescribed calcitonin 100 units IM. The drug on hand is 400 units/2 mL. How much should be administered?

26. A patient is prescribed heparin 25,000 units. The drug on hand is 1,000 units/mL. How much should be administered?

27. A patient is prescribed calcitonin 100 units IM. The drug on hand is 200 units/mL. How much should be administered?

28. A patient is prescribed heparin 25,000 units. The drug on hand is 10,000 units/mL. How much should be administered?

29. A patient is prescribed epoetin 38,000 units. The drug on hand is 4,000 units/mL. How much should be administered?

30. A patient is prescribed heparin 7,500 units SC. The drug on hand is 10,000 units/mL. How much should be administered?

31. A patient is prescribed heparin 5,000 units SC. The drug on hand is 10,000 units/mL. How much should be administered?

32. A patient is prescribed heparin 8,000 units SC. The drug on hand is 20,000 units/mL. How much should be administered?

33. A patient is prescribed 5,600 units of a medication. The drug on hand is 1,000 units/mL. How much should be administered?

34. A patient is prescribed 2,000 units of a medication. The drug on hand is 250 units/mL. How much should be administered?

35. A patient is prescribed calcitonin 250 units IM. The drug on hand is 400 units/2 mL. How much should be administered?

36. A patient is prescribed heparin 2,500 units. The drug on hand is 1,000 units/mL. How much should be administered?

37. A patient is prescribed calcitonin 150 units IM. The drug on hand is 200 units/mL. How much should be administered?

38. A patient is prescribed heparin 1,000 units. The drug on hand is 2,500 units/mL. How much should be administered?

39. A patient is prescribed epoetin 10,000 units. The drug on hand is 4,000 units/mL. How much should be administered?

40. A patient is prescribed epoetin 1,000 units. The drug on hand is 4,000 units/mL. How much should be administered?

PRACTICE EXERCISE 11D

Solve for the following questions. Return to Module 11 Screen 3.6 of the Online Course for answers.

1. When calculating a dosage for a 2-month-old baby who is 11 lbs., which method should be used?

2. Which of the following methods for pediatric dosage calculation uses the child's body weight?

3. A 2-month-old baby has an ear infection. The baby is prescribed azithromycin. The adult dosage is 500 mg. The baby is 11 lbs. How much should the baby take?

4. A 3-year-old girl is prescribed penicillin. She is 35 lbs. The adult dose for penicillin is 360 mg. Using Clark's rule, how much should she take?

5. A 3-year-old girl is prescribed penicillin. She is 35 lbs. The adult dose for penicillin is 360 mg. Using Young's rule, how much should she take?

Practice Drill 11D

Solve for the following problems. Answers to Practice Drills are found in the back of your workbook.

1. Which of the following pediatric dosage rule should be used if the child's weight is known?

2. Which of the following pediatric dosage rule should be used for children over one year, age is known but not body weight?

3. A 2-month-old baby has an ear infection. The baby is prescribed azithromycin. The adult dosage is 500 mg. The baby is 11 lbs. How much should the baby take?

4. A 3-year-old girl is prescribed penicillin. She is 35 lbs. The adult dose for penicillin is 360 mg. Using Clark's rule, how much should she take?

127

5. Using Clark's rule, what is the dose for a 12-year-old girl who weighs 31.7kg if the average adult dose is 500mg?

6. The average adult dose for a drug is 250mg. Using Clark's rule, what dose should be given to an 8-year-old child who weighs 57lbs?

7. A child weighs 40 lbs. and is 5 years old. The adult dose for a drug is 250 mg. What is the corrected dose for the child using Clark's Rule?

8. A 2-year-old child weights 11.4 kg. The adult dose to be prescribed is 125 mg. Calculate the correct dose for the child using Clark's Rule.

9. A 7-year-old child weighs 48 lbs. is prescribed a drug at 400 mg for an adult dose. What would be the appropriate dose for the child using Clark's Rule?

10. A 3-year-old girl is prescribed penicillin. She is 35 lbs. The adult dose for penicillin is 360 mg. Using Young's rule, how much should she take?

11. The pediatric dose for a 9-year-old child who weighs 63lbs. needs to be determined. You learn that the adult dose for the same drug is 200mg. Using Young's rule, what dose should the child be given?

12. A child weighs 40 lbs. and is 5 years old. The adult dose for a drug is 250 mg. What is the corrected dose for the child using Young's Rule?

13. A 2-year-old child weighs 10 kg. The adult dose for a drug that is to be prescribed is 80 mg. Calculate the appropriate dose for the child using Young's Rule.

14. A 2-year-old child weights 11.4 kg. The adult dose to be prescribed is 125 mg. Calculate the correct dose for the child using Young's Rule.

15. A 10-year-old girl who is 60 lbs. is prescribed 400 mg of an adult dose. What is the appropriate dose for this child?

16. Diphenhydramine 50 mg PO q6hr is prescribed to a 4-year-old child. Using Fried's Rule, what would be the dosage for the child?

17. An adult dose of a drug is 250 mg. Using Fried's Rule, what is the pediatric dose for a 3-year-old child?

18. An 18-month baby is prescribed amoxicillin. She is 42 lbs. The adult dosage is 40 mg. What would be dosage for the baby based on the Fried's rule?

19. A 5-year-old child is prescribed erythromycin. An adult dosage is 500 mg. What is the appropriate dosage for this child using Fried's rule?

20. Using Clark's rule, what is the dose for a 11-year-old boy who weighs 35.2 kg if the average adult dose is 400mg?

21. A 7-year-old pediatric patient is admitted to hospital. If the adult dose is 100 mg and the child weighs 40 kg, what dose should the child be administered if using the Young's rule?

A 10-year-old boy needs to be prescribed an antibacterial drug 35 mg. He weighs 32 kg. The adult dose for the same medicine is 75 mg. Calculate the boy's dosage using Clark's rule and Young's rules.

22. Clark's rule: _____

23. Young's rule: _____

A child weighs 40 lbs. and is 5 years old is prescribed a drug. The adult dose for the drug is 250 mg. Calculate the correct dose for the child using Young's and Clark's rules.

24. Clark's rule: _____

25. Young's rule: _____

A 2-year-old child that weighs 11.4 kg is prescribed a drug. The adult dose for this drug is 125 mg. Calculate the correct dose for the child using Young's and Clark's rules.

26. Clark's rule: _____

27. Young's rule: _____

An 18-month-old child is prescribed amoxicillin. She weighs 26 lbs. The adult dose is 500 mg. Calculate the correct dose for the child using Young's and Clark's rules.

28. Clark's rule: _____

29. Young's rule: _____

30. A child is prescribed Benedryl (diphenhydramine) 50 mg PO every 6 hours PRN. Calculate the dose for a 4-year-old child using Fried's Rule.

31. A child is prescribed morphine 2 mg IV every 4 hours PRN for pain. Calculate the dose for a 2½ year old child using Fried's Rule.

32. A child is prescribed Tylenol (acetaminophen) 500 mg PO PRN pain. Calculate the dose for a 7-year-old child using Young's Rule.

33. A child is prescribed an adult dose of Dilantin (phenytoin) 100 mg TID. Calculate the dose for a child weighing 25 lbs. using Clark's Rule.

34. A child is prescribed an adult dose of amoxicillin 500 mg q8h. Calculate the dose for a child weighing 18 lbs. using Clark's Rule.

35. A 2-year-old child weighs 10 kg. The adult dose for the drug to be used is 80 mg. Calculate the appropriate dose for the child using Young's Rule.

36. A 7-year-old child who weighs 48 lbs. requires a drug whose adult dose is 400 mg. What would be the correct dose for the child according to Clark's rule?

37. A 24-month-old child is prescribed ibuprofen. The adult dosage is 600 mg PO PRN. What would be the correct dose for the child according to Fried's rule?

38. A 5-year-old child is prescribe Lasix. The adult dosage is 20 mg PO. What would be the correct dose for the child according to Young's Rule?

39. A child is prescribed an adult dose of 2 million units of penicillin G potassium per day divided into 4 doses. Calculate the dose per day for a 10-year-old child using Young's Rule.

40. A 10-month-old child is prescribed Decadron (dexamethasone). The patient weight 16 lbs. The adult dosage is 4 mg/day. Calculate the dose using Clark's Rule.

REVIEW EXERCISES

Using the methods in this module, solve for the following problems. Answers to Review Exercises are found in the back of your workbook.

1. A person weighs 185 lbs. and is prescribed 1.5 mg/kg of a drug. What is the dosage?

2. A person weighs 215 lbs. and is prescribed 0.25 mL/kg. How much should be administered?

3. A patient weights 200 lbs. Aspirin is prescribed for 300 mg. The drug label shows the dosage strength to be 65 mg/kg. What is the dosage?

4. A medication order is for amoxicillin 200 mg PO BID. The amoxicillin on hand is 400 mg/5 mL. How much should you administer?

5. A medication order is for erythromycin 500 mg PO BID. The drug label shows the dosage strength as 400 mg/5 mL. How much should you administer?

6. Humalog (U-100) is an injectable insulin. Each cartridge is 3 mL and contains 100 units of Humalog. The medication order is for 17 units. How much should you administer? (Use Fig. 11.12.)

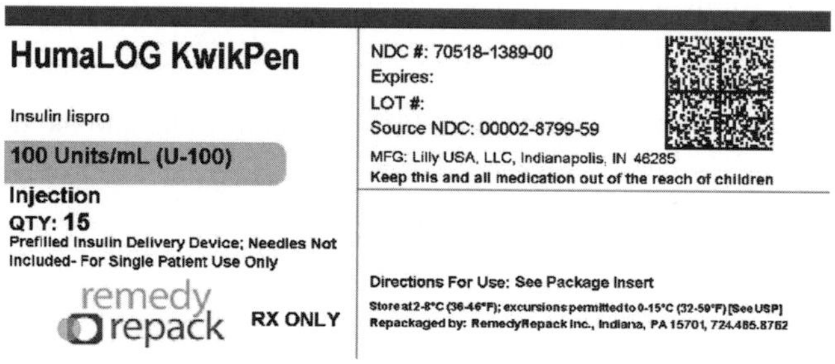

HumaLOG KwikPen

Insulin lispro

100 Units/mL (U-100)

Injection
QTY: 15
Prefilled Insulin Delivery Device; Needles Not
Included- For Single Patient Use Only

remedy repack   **RX ONLY**

NDC #: 70518-1389-00
Expires:
LOT #:
Source NDC: 00002-8799-59
MFG: Lilly USA, LLC, Indianapolis, IN 46285
Keep this and all medication out of the reach of children

Directions For Use: See Package Insert
Store at 2-8°C (36-46°F); excursions permitted to 9-15°C (32-59°F) [See USP]
Repackaged by: RemedyRepack Inc., Indiana, PA 15701, 724.485.8762

Figure 11.12

A patient weights 122 lbs. Ampicillin is prescribed for 500 mg every 6 hours. The dosage strength is 125 mg/5 mL.

7. What is this patient's weight in kg.?

8. How much should be administered each time?

9. How many mg of ampicillin does the patient take each day?

Use the drug label in Fig. 11.13 to answer Questions #10-13.

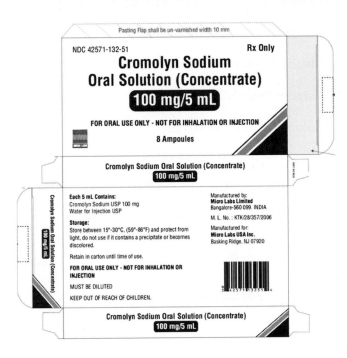

Figure 11.13

A physician prescribes cromolyn sodium as part of a patient's asthma treatment. The medication order is for 20 mg QID. The patient is 7 years old and weights 56 lbs.

10. What is the total dosage of the drug each day?

11. What is the dosage using Clark's rule?

12. What is the dosage using Young's rule?

13. The prescribed dose for the child is 7.5 mg of cromolyn sodium. How much should be administered each time?

Use the drug label in Fig. 11.14 to answer Questions #14-16.

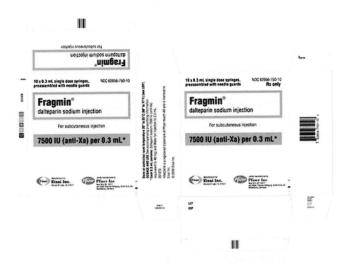

Figure 11.14

Module **11** Weight-Based Dosage Calculations

Fragmin (dalteparin) is an anticoagulant used in heart conditions and to prevent blood clots. The dosage strength on hand is 7,500 IU per 0.3 mL. The recommended dosage is 120 IU/kg every 12 hours. The patient weights 250 lbs.

14. What is the dosage (IU) the patient should be taking each time?

15. What is the total amount of drug in the entire package of Fragmin?

16. What is the patient's daily dosage of Fragmin?

Use the drug label in Fig. 11.15 to answer Questions #17-20.

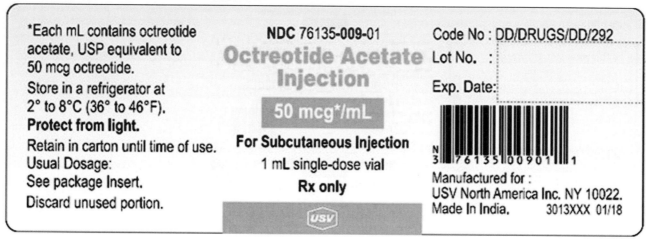

Figure 11.15

The medication order is for 75 mcg SC every 12 hours.

17. How much of the drug is contained in this vial?

18. How much should you prepare for each injection?

19. Based on the medication order, what is the patient's daily dosage?

20. The recommended dosage of octreotide acetate is 300 mcg/day. How many mL of drug is this per day?

A patient is 132 lbs. The drug dose ordered is 1.4 mg/kg per day QID.

21. How much of the drug should the patient receive per day?

22. How much of the drug should the patient receive per dose?

A patient is 36 lbs. The dose ordered for the drug is 0.5 mg/kg PRN q6h.

23. How much of the drug should the patient receive per day?

24. How much of the drug should the patient receive per dose?

A patient is 212 lbs. The dose ordered for the drug is 0.25 mg/kg every 8 hours.

25. How much of the drug should the patient receive per day?

26. How much of the drug should the patient receive per dose?

27. A patient is 22 lbs. The drug is ordered at 0.5 mcg/kg every 6 hours. How much of the drug should the patient receive per day?

28. Cephalosporin is ordered for a child whose weight is 35 lbs. The recommended dose is 50 mg/kg. What is the daily dose?

29. Ampicillin is prescribed to a 10 lb. infant at 125 mg/kg. How much should be administered?

30. A 20 lb. child is prescribed morphine 0.5 mg/kg IM. How much should be administered?

A child weighs 55 lbs. She is prescribed carbamazepine 400 mg PO BID. The safe dosage is 15 mg/kg – 20 mg/kg.

31. How much should be administered?

32. Is the prescribed dosage within the recommended dosage range?

Erythromycin is prescribed 62.5 mg PO q6hr for a 11-lb infant. The safe dosage should not exceed 50 mg/kg/24 hrs.

33. What is the daily dosage?

34. What is the maximum dosage this child may receive of erythromycin?

35. Is the prescribe dosage for the infant within the safe dosage range?

Acetaminophen is prescribed 10 mg/kg PO. The child is 10 lbs. Acetaminophen on hand is 160 mg/5 mL.

36. How much acetaminophen should be administered to the child?

37. How many mL should the child receive?

Amoxicillin is prescribed 200 mg PO BID. The child weighs 15 lbs. Amoxicillin should not exceed 30 mg/kg/24 hours.

38. What is the ordered dose for the child per day?

39. What is the maximum daily dosage?

40. Is the ordered dosage safe?

41. Phenytoin is prescribed 8 mg/kg/24 hours. The child weight 30 lb. How much should be administered per day?

42. Digoxin is prescribed 18 mcg PO BID. The child weighs 7 lb. The safe dosage should not exceed 12 mcg/kg/24 hours. Is what is prescribed below the safe dosage?

43. Breylium 5 mcg/kg/min is prescribed to a 187 lb patient. How much should be administered to the patient in milligrams?

44. An infant weights 8 lbs. and is prescribed 15 mg/kg of a drug. What is the dosage?

45. A child weights 18 lbs. and is prescribed 0.25 mL/kg. What is the dosage?

Use the drug label in Fig. 11.16 to answer Questions #46-50.

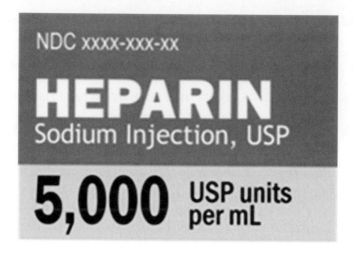

NDC xxxx-xxx-xx

HEPARIN
Sodium Injection, USP

5,000 USP units
per mL

For IV or SC use
Rx only

10 mL
Multiple Dose Vial

Figure 11.16

46. Based on the drug label, how can heparin be administered?

47. How much heparin is in 1 mL?

48. How much heparin is contained in the vial?

49. The medication order is for heparin 15,000 IU SC BID. What is the dosage of heparin the patient will be administered every day?

50. A medication order is for the patient to receive heparin 8,000 IU SC every 8 hours. How many mL of heparin does he receive daily?

12 Basic Statistics in Healthcare

INTRODUCTION TO BASIC STATISTICS

Practice Exercise 12A

Solve for the following questions. Return to Module 12 Screen 1.4 of the Online Course for answers.

1. Calculate the mean of 8, 15, and 22.

2. Calculate the mean of 55, 72, 85, 155, and 210.

3. A seminar had the following number of people attend each session: 854, 1210, and 1285. On average, how many people attended a session?

4. You are weighing your patient as part of his check-in. What is his average weight over the last six months?

Month	Weight (lbs.)
January	205
February	205
March	206
April	207
May	204
June	199

5. Your medical office is ordering supplies for the next month. To know how much to order, what is the average number of boxes gloves does the office use each month?

Month	Boxes
June	12
July	15
August	11
September	14
October	16
November	18

Practice Drills 12A

Solve for the following questions. Round to the nearest tenths place. Answers to Practice Drills are found in the back of your workbook.

1. Calculate the mean of 10, 15, and 20.

2. Calculate the mean of 6, 7, and 11.

3. What is the mean of the numbers 8, 9, 13 and 18?

4. Calculate the mean of 155, 172, 185, 255, and 1,210.

5. What number would you divide by to calculate the mean of 3, 4, 5, and 6?

6. What number would you divide by to calculate the mean of 68, 55, 70, 62, 71, 58, 81, 82, 63, and 73?

7. What number would you divide by to calculate the mean of the data in Table 12.1?

Month	Weight (lbs.)
January	205
February	205
March	206
April	207
May	204
June	199

Table 12.1

8. What is the mean of 59, 20, 106, 36, and 52?

9. What is the mean of 10, 39, 71, 42, 39, 76, 38, and 25?

10. What is the mean of 43, 37, 35, 30, 41, 23, 33, 31, 16, and 21.

11. What is the mean of 3, −7, 5, 13, and −2?

12. What is the mean of 68, 55, 70, 62, 71, 58, 81, 82, 63, and 73?

Subject	Grade
Math	51%
English	62%
Science	70%
Geography	39%
History	81%
Economics	57%

Table 12.2

13. A student receives his report card. What is the average grade for his courses (Use Table 12.2)?

14. The scores on an exam are: 90, 50, 70, 80, 70, 60, 20, 30, 80, 90, and 20. What is the average score on the exam?

Calculate the mean for the following data sets.

15. 3, 9, 13, 8, 10, 2

16. 3, 6, 10, 5, 16, 3, 6

17. 10, 9, 10, 11, 13, 13, 5

18. 9, 15, 1, 19, 4, 6

19. 2, 19, 4, 1, 8

20. 10, 12, 6, 1, 9, 16, 20, 17, 8

21. 2, 11, 5, 6, 13, 4, 9

22. 9, 12, 20, 16, 7, 20

23. 7, 14, 10, 19, 9, 17, 16

24. 12, 3, 14, 18, 2, 5, 9

25. 10, 13, 11, 10, 5, 9

26. 18, 11, 10, 8, 9, 5, 9, 10

27. 19, 1, 18, 17, 9, 7, 6, 10, 1

28. 11, 17, 4, 13, 20, 10, 16

29. 18, 19, 11, 17, 5, 19

30. 9, 7, 11, 13, 2, 4, 5, 5

31. 23, 23, 27, 29, 29, 35

32. 40, 61, 95, 79, 9, 50, 80, 63, 109, 42

33. 3, 7, 5, 13, 20, 23, 39, 23, 40, 23, 14, 12, 56, 23, 29

34. 62 kg, 63 kg, 62 kg, 57 kg

35. 12, -1, 8, 2, -10, 0, -5, 3, 20, -2

Solve for the following questions.

36. The mean weight of five people is 167.2 pounds. The weights of four people are 158.4 pounds, 162.8 pounds, 165 pounds, and 178.2 pounds. What is the weight of the fifth person?

37. The mean weight of a group of seven boys is 56 lbs. The individual weights of six of them are 52 lbs., 57 lbs., 55 lbs., 60 lbs., 59 lbs., and 55 lbs. What is the weight of the seventh boy?

38. The mean of 8, 11, 6, 14, χ, and 13 is 66. Find the value of the observation χ.

137

39. The mean of four numbers is 71.5. If three of the numbers are 58, 76, and 88, what is the value of the fourth number?

40. The mean of 6, 8, x + 2, 10, 2x - 1, and 2 is 9. Find the value of x.

Practice Exercise 12B

Identify the median in the following data sets. Return to Module 12 Screen 1.7 of the Online Course for answers.

1. {7, 9, 3, 2, 1, 3, 4}

2. {17, 8, 15, 21, 12}

3. $110, $12, $56, $3, $102, $8, $99

4. {17, 8, 15, 21, 12, 15}

5. $110, $12, $56, $3, $102, $8, $99, $15

Practice Drills 12B

Identify the median in the following data sets. Round to the nearest tenths place. Answers to Practice Drills are found in the back of your workbook.

1. 5, 7, 8, 2 and 4

2. 16, 24, 8, 12, and 19

3. 15, 32, 53, 27, and 11

4. 75, 29, 12, 17, and 15

5. 142, 173, 129, 156, and 181

6. 257, 366, 305, 286, and 182

7. 82, 106, 91, 115, 78, 83, and 102

8. 428, 417, 472, 456, and 409

9. 3, 19, 26, 3, 8, 37, 12, 5, and 0

10. 819, 862, 851, 904, and 786

11. 8, −2, 0, 4, and 7

12. 10, 6, and −3

13. 0, 7, 2, 5, and −1

14. 6, −5, 4, −2, and 3

15. 3, −6, −2, −5, 0, 1, and −2

16. 73, 27, 46, 108, 9, 63, and 4

17. −14, −6, −10, −3, and −12

18. 6, −2, −8, 0, 2, −1, −5, 2, and −2

19. 1.5, 0.7, 2.3, 1.1, and 3.8

20. 1.8, 0.7, and 1.1

21. 4.2, 6.1, 3.5, 2.2, and 4.6

22. 2.5, 3.1, 1.7, and 4.8

23. 3, 1.8, 2, and 4.7

24. 0.3, 1.5, 0.7, 1.2, 0.3, and 1.1

25. 5.8, 2.7, 3.1, 1.9, 9, and 2.3

26. 5.16, 4.9, 5.7, 4.32, and 5.65

27. 4.39, 4.2, 3.98, 4.8, and 3.7

28. 214, 209, 243, and 226

29. 4, −9, −3, −5, 7, 8, and −5, 8

Solve for the following questions.

30. The ages of children in a family are 3, 7, 10, and 12

31. The salaries of the hospital staff are:
    $127,950
    $34,725
    $102,465
    $99,100
    $45,617
    $78,125

32. An instructor wants to know the distribution of an exam. The students' grades are:
    99, 77, 69, 97, 88, 82, 91, 74

33. A home health aide wants to know the range of miles she has to drive to see visit each of her patients.
    Patient 1: 25 miles
    Patient 2: 45 miles
    Patient 3: 12 miles
    Patient 4: 15 miles
    Patient 5: 22 miles

34. What is the median of 5, 7, 4, 9, 5, 4, 4, and 3?

35. What is the median of the following data: 25, 20, 30, 30, 20, 24, 24, 30, and 31?

36. What is the median of the following data: 1, 6, 12, 19, 5, 0, and 6?

37. What is the median of the following data: 9, 6, 12, 5, 17, 3, 9, 5, 10, 2, 8, and 7?

139

38. What is the median of the data 23, 49, 87, 75, 88, 59, and 89?

39. Calculate the median in the following data set.
{22, 16, 14, 24, 11, 10}

40. On an exam, students can score 1 to 100. What is the median exam score?

Practice Exercise 12C

Calculate the range. Return to Module 12 Screen 1.12 of the Online Course for answers.

1. 6, 52, 10, 15, 27, and 4

2. The ages of children in a family are 3, 7, 10, and 12

3. The salaries of the hospital staff are:
$127,950
$34,725
$102,465
$99,100
$45,617
$78,125

4. An instructor wants to know the distribution of an exam. The students' grades are:
99, 77, 69, 97, 88, 82, 91, and 74

5. A home health aide wants to know the range of miles she has to drive to see visit each of her patients.
Patient 1: 25 miles
Patient 2: 45 miles
Patient 3: 12 miles
Patient 4: 15 miles
Patient 5: 22 miles

Practice Drills 12C

Answer the following questions. Answers to Practice Drills are found in the back of your workbook.

1. What is the mode of the following numbers: 12, 11, 14, 10, 8, 13, 11, and 9?

2. What is the mode of the following sets of numbers: 3, 13, 6, 8, 10, 5, and 6?

3. What is the mode of the following sets of numbers: 12, 0, 15, 15, 13, 19, 16, 13, 16, and 16?

4. The front row in a movie theatre has 23 seats. If you were asked to sit in the seat that occupied the median position, in which seat would you have to sit?

5. What is the mode of the following data: 20, 14, 12, 14, 26, 16, 18, 19, and 14?

6. What is the mode of the following data: 5, 0, 5, 4, 12, 2, and 14?

7. What is the mode of the data 21, 26, 22, 29, 23, 29, 26, 29, 22, and 23?

Use the following data set to answer Questions #5-7.
Jessica scores the following on her last seven exams: 70, 80, 70, 90, 80, 70, and 100. What is the mode and range of her exam scores?

8. Mode: _____

   Range: _____

A patient has diabetes and his hemoglobin A1C levels must be checked every 3 months. They are as follows:

January	8.0
April	7.5
July	8.0
October	8.5
December	9.5

9. What is the mode and range of the patient's results?

   Mode: _____

   Range: _____

Calculate the median for the following data set.

10. 19, 9, 16, 4, 4, 19, 1, 20, and 6

11. 6, 19, 2, 14, 9, 18, 14, 14, and 11

12. 12, 16, 17, 17, 4, 17, and 4

13. 7, 2, 6, 17, 14, 4, 20, and 5

14. 19, 11, 7, 12, 17, 4, 20, and 19

15. 20, 11, 19, 20, 16, and 5

16. 13, 10, 7, 19, 12, 1, 15, 5, and 1

17. 18, 2, 7, 20, 9, 3, 11, and 3

Calculate the mode for the following data set.

18. 65, 56, 52, 57, 60, 53, 53, 52, 67, and 52

19. 85, 91, 83, 79, 77, 80, 91, 75, 87, and 91

20. 21, 23, 37, 30, 21, 36, 26, 33, 27, 41, 27, and 21

21. 95, 79, 88, 86, 98, 95, 87, and 92

22. 25, 12, 24, 25, 22, 16, 15, 17, 26, 10, and 16

23. 29, 28, 20, 24, 30, 20, 40, 23, 33, 36, and 36

24. 51, 60, 52, 58, 66, 53, 54, 60, 52, and 51

Calculate the mode and range for the following data set.

25. 15, 23, 19, 20, and 23

Mode: _____

Range: _____

26. 22, 37, 19, 25, 37, 51, and 82

Mode: _____

Range: _____

27. 2, 7, 4, 2, 3, 6, and 11

Mode: _____

Range: _____

28. 6, 2, 13, 7, 6, 11, 10, 6, and 2

Mode: _____

Range: _____

29. 70, 63, 67, 62, and 63

Mode: _____

Range: _____

30. 109, 104, 96, 103, 104, 107, and 98

Mode: _____

Range: _____

31. 11, 4, 7, 8, 2, 6, and 4

Mode: _____

Range: _____

32. 14, 68, 38, 65, 36, 57, and 65

Mode: _____

Range: _____

33. 32, 37, 35, 34, 25, 41, and 34

Mode: _____

Range: _____

34. 126, 128, 107, 113, 120, and 126

Mode: _____

Range: _____

35. 102, 107, 99, 102, 111, 95, and 91

   Mode: _____

   Range: _____

36. 5.2, 4.9, 3.8, 3.4, 5.2, and 4.5

   Mode: _____

   Range: _____

37. 1.5, 2.2, 1.3, 2.8, and 2.2

   Mode: _____

   Range: _____

38. 0.24, 0.5, 0.09, 0.73, and 0.24

   Mode: _____

   Range: _____

39. 2.9, 4.3, 3.5, 5.8, 2.9, and 5.8

   Mode: _____

   Range: _____

40. 116, 130, 120, 125, 140, and 125

   Mode: _____

   Range: _____

REVIEW EXERCISES

Using the methods in this chapter, solve for the following problems. Return to the online course to review any content. Answers to Review Exercises are found in the back of your workbook.

1. Which of the following is the middle value of a data set?
   a. Mean
   b. Median
   c. Mode
   d. Range

2. To determine the average of a set of numbers is called the _____.
   a. Mean
   b. Median
   c. Mode
   d. Range

3. When you add all the values and divide by the number of values, this will be the _____.
   a. Mean
   b. Median
   c. Mode
   d. Range

4. The _____ is the value most occurring in a data set.
   a. Mean
   b. Median
   c. Mode
   d. Range

5. Which of the following is <u>not</u> a measure of central tendency?
   a. Mean
   b. Median
   c. Mode
   d. Range

6. Which of the following is calculated based on taking the difference between the highest and lowest number in the data set?
   a. Mean
   b. Median
   c. Mode
   d. Range

Use Table 12.3 to answer Questions #7-10.
The table below shows the results from an exam.

Student	Exam Score
Christia	89
Dakota	85
Blanche	77
Nina	92
Portia	80
Lasonya	85

Table 12.3

7. What is the mean of the exam results?

8. What is the median of the exam results?

9. What is the mode of the exam results?

10. What is the range of the exam results?

Use Table 12.4 to answer Questions #11-18.
The table below shows the exam results from two classes.

Mrs. Curtis		Mr. Barr	
Student	Score	Student	Score
Ping	94	Alex	91
Louis	65	Rose	88
Bryan	80	Fatimah	94
Lin	78	Juan	79
Sherron	72	Lucien	88
Sonia	88	David	95

Table 12.4

144

11. What is the mean of the exam results in Mrs. Curtis' class?

12. What is the mean of the exam results in Mr. Barr's class?

13. Both classes took the same exam. What is the mode of the exam?

14. What is the median of Mrs. Curtis' class?

15. What is the median of Mr. Barr's class?

16. What is the range of Mrs. Curtis' class?

17. What is the range of Mr. Barr's class?

18. Whose class had the lowest distribution of exam scores?

Use the following data set for Questions #19-22.
   13, 13, 13, 15, 16, 16, and 16

19. What is the mode?

20. What is the mean?

21. What is the median?

22. What is the range?

Use the following data set for Questions #23-26.
   20, 20, 20, 40, 40, 70, and 80

23. What is the mode?

24. What is the mean?

25. What is the median?

26. What is the range?

Use the following data set to answer Questions #27-29.
Alice started a weight loss program. Her initial weight is 160 lbs. Over the course of the next several weeks, her weight has been 156 lbs., 148.5 lbs. 150 lbs., 147 lbs., 142 lbs., and 138 lbs.

27. What is Alice's median weight?

28. What is the range?

29. What is Alice's average weight loss?

Use the following data set to answer Questions #30-34.
Ryan scores the following on his history exam: 75, 81, 92, 75, 86, 90, and 75.

30. What is the median?

31. What is the mode?

32. What is the range?

33. What is the mean?

34. If Ryan wants to increase the average score, what is the minimum score he will need on his next exam?

Use Table 12.5 to answer Questions #35-40.

Students	Exam Scores
Ann	71, 64, 63, 77, 80, 79, and 80
Mimi	90, 92, 96, 99, 99, 89, and 97
Brian	100, 100, 100, 100, 100, 100, and 100
Wendy	83, 89, 80, 82, 89, 79, and 79
Sandra	63, 61, 66, 66, 70, 71, and 65

Table 12.5

35. What is the median of Ann's scores?

36. What is the mode of Mimi's scores?

37. What is the range of Brian's scores?

38. Which student has the lowest average exam score?

39. Which student has the highest average exam score?

40. If everyone scored 100 on the next exam, whose average score would increase the most?

Calculate the mean, median, mode, and range for the following data sets.

41.   83, 93, 77, 33, 62, 28, and 23
      Mean: _____
      Median: _____
      Mode: _____
      Range: _____

42. 31, 92, 25, 69, 80, 31, and 29

    Mean: _____

    Median: _____

    Mode: _____

    Range: _____

43. 86, 13, 60, 55, 61, 97, 30, 98, 79, 52, and 18

    Mean: _____

    Median: _____

    Mode: _____

    Range: _____

44. 24, 22, 32, 59, 99, 59, 76, 83, 21, 95, and 57

    Mean: _____

    Median: _____

    Mode: _____

    Range: _____

45. 63, 25, 43, 28, 72, 61, 45, 46, and 13

    Mean: _____

    Median: _____

    Mode: _____

    Range: _____

46. 83, 23, 24, 71, 52, 62, and 63

    Mean: _____

    Median: _____

    Mode: _____

    Range: _____

47. 53, 44, 10, 45, 59, 97, and 77

    Mean: _____

    Median: _____

    Mode: _____

    Range: _____

48. 82, 23, 59, 94, 70, 26, 32, 83, 87, 94, and 32

    Mean: _____

    Median: _____

    Mode: _____

    Range: _____

49. 21, 62, 66, 66, 79, 28, 63, 48, 59, 94, and 19

Mean: _____

Median: _____

Mode: _____

Range: _____

50. 1211, 2916, 471, 1211, and 5045

Mean: _____

Median: _____

Mode: _____

Range: _____

Post-Assessment

Solve for the following problems. Answers to the Post-Assessment are found in the back of your workbook.

1. $876 - 18$

2. Solve for x.

    $512 + x + 12 = 850$

3. 134×11

4. $324 \div 26$

5. $952 \div 1.7$

6. $130.5 \div 2.1$

7. Order the following from smallest to largest: $\frac{10}{11}, \frac{1}{2}, \frac{1}{16}$.

8. $11 + 30\frac{3}{5} + 3\frac{1}{3}$

9. $15 + (15 \div 3) - 10$

10. $\frac{3}{7} \times 2 \times 2\frac{9}{10}$

11. $11\frac{2}{3} \div 2\frac{5}{6}$

12. Convert 10:12 PM to 24-hour time.

13. Convert 3:30 AM to 24-hour time.

14. Convert 00:45 to 12-hour time.

15. Convert 100.2°F to °C.

16. Convert 22°C to °F.

17. 5 mg = _____ g

18. 11.7 kg = _____ g

19. 0.198 g = _____ mcg

20. 75.36 mg = _____ mcg

21. Convert 2,685,321.15 mcg = _____ kg. Round to the nearest hundredth place.

A patient's temperature is taken over several days. Use the following table for Questions #22-24.

Day 1	99.8°F
Day 2	99.8°F
Day 3	101.1°F
Day 4	100.3°F
Day 5	100.0°F
Day 6	99.0°F
Day 7	98.8°F

22. What is the mean of the patient's temperatures?

23. What is the mode of the patient's temperatures?

24. What is the range of the patient's temperatures?

25. A patient is 5' 2" tall and weighs 125 lbs. What is her height in inches?

26. A patient is 5' 2" tall and weighs 125 lbs. What is her height in meters?

27. A patient is 5' 2" tall and weighs 125 lbs. What is her weight in kg?

Pamelor (nortriptyline) is a prescription medication often used to treat depression. Use the drug label shown below to answer Questions #28-31.

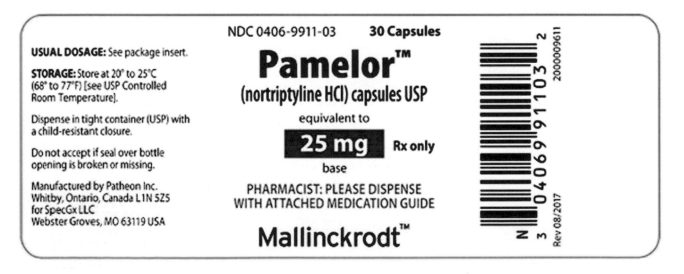

28. What is the brand name of this drug?

29. What is the dosage on hand?

30. What is the quantity on hand?

31. If the patient is prescribed to take 4 capsules a day, what is the patient's daily dosage?

Cleocin (clindamycin) is an antibiotic used to treat several types of bacterial infections, such as pharyngitis, tonsilitis, and otitis media (ear infections). Use the drug label shown below to answer Questions #32-35.

NDC 0009-0331-02

Cleocin HCl®

clindamycin hydrochloride capsules, USP

75 mg*

100 Capsules   Rx only

Store at controlled room temperature 20° to 25° C (68° to 77° F) [see USP]. DOSAGE AND USE: See accompanying prescribing information.
* Each capsule contains clindamycin hydrochloride equivalent to 75 mg of clindamycin.
2000012013

MADE IN CANADA
Distributed by Pharmacia & Upjohn Co Division of Pfizer Inc, NY, NY 10017

32. What is the generic name of the drug?

33. What is the dosage strength?

34. What is the quantity on hand?

35. The patient is prescribed 150 mg PO QID. How many capsules will the patient receive each day?

Use the drug label shown below to answer Questions #36-38.

*Each mL contains octreotide acetate, USP equivalent to 50 mcg octreotide.
Store in a refrigerator at 2° to 8°C (36° to 46°F). **Protect from light.**
Retain in carton until time of use.
Usual Dosage: See package Insert.
Discard unused portion.

NDC 76135-009-01
Octreotide Acetate Injection
50 mcg*/mL
For Subcutaneous Injection
1 mL single-dose vial
Rx only
USV

Code No : DD/DRUGS/DD/292
Lot No. :
Exp. Date:

N 3 76135 00901 1

Manufactured for :
USV North America Inc. NY 10022.
Made In India.   3013XXX 01/18

36. What is the route of administration?

37. What is the dosage on hand?

38. The patient is prescribed octreotide 0.3 mg SC TID. How much should be administered each time?

Use the drug label shown below to answer Questions #39-42.

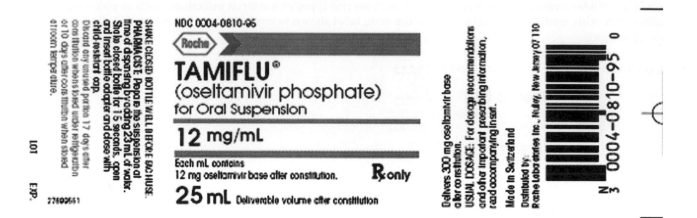

39. What is the quantity on hand?

40. What is total amount of the drug in the vial?

41. The patient is prescribed 75 mg PO BID for 5 days. How many milliliters should the patient take every day?

42. Tamiflu may be prescribed to children. The recommended pediatric dosage for children between 1-12 years of age is based on body weight. The child is prescribed 75 mg PO QD. How much should be administered to a 70 lb. child?

Acyclovir is a prescription medication used as a topical, injectable, and oral treatment for genital herpes and cold sores. Use the drug label shown below to answer Questions #43-47.

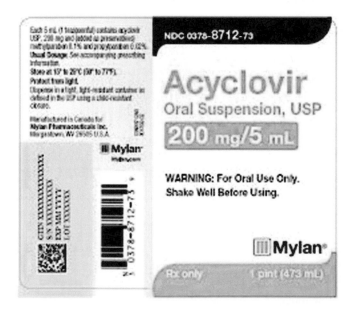

43. What is the dosage strength per mL?

44. The patient is prescribed 400 mg of acyclovir PO every 4 hours. How much should the patient be administered each time?

45. What is the patient's daily dosage of acyclovir?

46. What would be the pediatric dosage for an 8-year-old child receiving the same adult dosage of 400 mg?

47. How much should be administered to the 8-year-old child?

A patient is prescribed a drug at 15 mg/kg per day. The dosage on hand is 750 mg/5 mL. The patient weights 228 lbs.

48. How much does the patient weight in kilograms? (Round to the nearest hundredth place.)

49. What is the medication dosage the patient should be receiving each day?

50. How much should be administered?

Answer Key

1. 7
2. 5
3. 7
4. 7
5. 100.1678
6. 8
7. 14
8. XXVI
9. 5
10. 7
11. 155
12. 251
13. 53
14. 950.9
15. 1.8
16. 224
17. 4,160
18. 0.378
19. 42
20. 210
21. 115
22. 102
23. $\frac{5}{8}$
24. $5\frac{1}{3}$
25. $1\frac{4}{5}$
26. $\frac{22}{5}$
27. $\frac{1}{5}$
28. $\frac{1}{5}$
29. $1\frac{11}{20}$
30. $4\frac{11}{12}$
31. $\frac{1}{4}$
32. $2\frac{7}{12}$
33. $\frac{2}{5}$
34. $\frac{9}{10}$
35. $4\frac{1}{2}$
36. $3\frac{3}{5}$
37. $\frac{3}{20}$
38. $7\frac{1}{5}$
39. 1.713
40. 80.2
41. 0.655
42. 1.25
43. $\frac{1}{5}$
44. $2\frac{3}{4}$
45. $x = 4$
46. $x = 16$
47. $x = 9$
48. $4,784
49. 3 teaspoons of salt
50. $2\frac{1}{2}$ pizzas

Answer Key

Practice Drills 1A

1. 2
2. 0
3. 718986
4. 11
5. 10
6. tens
7. ones
8. thousands
9. hundred thousands
10. millions
11. −17
12. 0
13. 130
14. 99
15. −5
16. 4
17. −515
18. −11
19. 135
20. 0
21. 6
22. 50
23. 8
24. 12
25. −5
26. 12
27. 2
28. 10
29. 4
30. 12

Practice Drills 1B

1. 13
2. 15
3. 33
4. 4
5. 22
6. 24
7. 22
8. 16
9. 37
10. 29
11. III or iii
12. V
13. IX or ix
14. XVII or xvii
15. XXVII or xxvii
16. XII or xii
17. XXXIX or xxxix
18. XIV or xiv
19. XXXIV or xxxiv
20. XXVIII or xxviii
21. XXXIII or xxxiii
22. XIX or xix
23. X or x
24. XII or xii
25. XXI or xxi
26. XXXVI or xxxvi
27. XXXI or xxxi
28. XX
29. XXVII or xxvii
30. XV or xv
31. 22
32. 16
33. 3
34. 28
35. 14
36. 8
37. 19
38. 7
39. 14
40. 32

Practice Drills 1C

1. XL
2. XC
3. CD
4. CXX
5. CML
6. LVIII
7. CCXL
8. DXIV
9. CDIV
10. MMCL
11. 51
12. 110
13. 116
14. 55
15. 1,001
16. 499
17. 999

18. 89
19. 99
20. 474
21. 82
22. 101
23. 701
24. 54
25. 66
26. 73
27. 90
28. 1,003
29. 535
30. 49
31. CDXXXIII
32. DXXX
33. L
34. XCIII
35. DL
36. 68
37. 1,500
38. 602
39. 456
40. 313

Chapter 1 Review Exercises

1. ones
2. hundreds
3. hundreds
4. ones
5. ten thousands
6. millions
7. 17
8. 44
9. 0
10. 3,425
11. B. 5
12. D. 0
13. B. 5
14. C. −7
15. A. 1.2
16. A. +152
17. 11
18. 9
19. 51
20. 1,500
21. 17
22. 33
23. 49
24. 38
25. 34
26. 130
27. 155
28. 162
29. 142

30. 79
31. 97
32. 153
33. 67
34. VIII
35. XII
36. XIX
37. XLIII
38. XXVIII
39. XV
40. LIV
41. XXXVIII
42. XC
43. LXXXVI
44. DCCCXC
45. CLIII
46. DCCXLII
47. DCCXXXVIII
48. DCLXXII
49. DLVI
50. CMLXXIV

CHAPTER 2

Practice Drills 2A

1. 15
2. 20
3. 83
4. 91
5. 79
6. 155
7. 165
8. 630
9. 482
10. 278
11. 265
12. 735
13. 758
14. 900
15. 1,434
16. 850
17. 980
18. 11,262
19. 1,677
20. 7,181
21. 2,435
22. 555
23. 2,200
24. 11,827
25. 6,476
26. 4,779
27. 62,424
28. 124,137
29. 11,691

30. 872,336
31. 50 pieces of candy
32. 86 shells
33. 982 attend the school
34. $1,050
35. $4,635
36. 162,855 is the total population of the city
37. 9,997 people
38. 4,270 miles
39. 18,615 crates
40. 3,489,000 people

Practice Drills 2B
1. 7
2. 15
3. 17
4. 27
5. 96
6. 506
7. 52
8. 11
9. 32
10. 26
11. 11
12. 202
13. 235
14. 2,249
15. 398
16. 96
17. 4,234
18. 3,604
19. 2,058
20. −77
21. 34
22. 500
23. 288
24. 676
25. -51
26. 908
27. −8
28. 331
29. 3,551
30. 2,999
31. 39
32. 449
33. 35,919
34. 12,121
35. 2,569
36. 46 coins
37. 137 tickets
38. 20,963 people
39. 2,598
40. 21,502

Chapter 2 Review Exercises
1. 7
2. 16
3. 12
4. 78
5. 11
6. 24
7. 17
8. 74
9. 90
10. 64
11. 71
12. 532
13. 306
14. 261
15. 758
16. 202
17. 235
18. 441
19. 293
20. 96
21. 398
22. 3,903
23. 2,249
24. 257
25. 9,821
26. 4,234
27. 1,679
28. 33,653
29. 876
30. 455
31. 1,032
32. 4,945
33. 2,664
34. 498
35. 2,492
36. 488
37. 2,215
38. 3,219
39. 3,604
40. 10,366
41. 60,523
42. 59,672
43. 96,249
44. 2,058
45. −77
46. 210
47. 4,340
48. 74,782
49. 42,146
50. −12,896

Practice Drills 3A

1. 2×3
2. 4×2
3. 1×5
4. 6×4
5. 8×3
6. 3×4
7. 10×4
8. 6
9. 8
10. 5
11. 24
12. 24
13. 12
14. 40
15. 28
16. 88
17. 630
18. 48
19. 88
20. 36
21. 39
22. 60
23. 18
24. 16
25. 15
26. 14
27. 30
28. 44
29. 36
30. 90
31. 27
32. 121
33. 48
34. 20
35. 10 pieces of candy
36. 16 slices
37. 14 pairs of socks
38. 100 books
39. 84 pill bottles
40. 60 patients

Practice Drills 3B

1. 39
2. 50
3. 77
4. 180
5. 630
6. 140
7. 408
8. 250
9. 3,050

10. 561
11. 1,284
12. 666
13. 2,400
14. 1,233
15. 1,066
16. 2,844
17. 24,966
18. 16,048
19. 14,707
20. 80,828
21. 615
22. 1,953
23. 7,424
24. 2,106
25. 1,626
26. 5,136
27. 2,195
28. 4,767
29. 1,888
30. 1,701
31. 7,788
32. 49,960
33. 27,896
34. 14,268
35. 6,120
36. 122,508
37. 31,276
38. 89,950
39. 732,920
40. 695,043

Practice Drills 3C

1. 48
2. 96
3. 435
4. 576
5. 32,445
6. 10,752
7. 936
8. 13,651
9. 4,152
10. 5,103
11. 4,094
12. 23,508
13. 96,900
14. 92,656
15. 648,288
16. 35,190
17. 568,945
18. 2,023,461
19. 226,152
20. 8,204,350
21. 2,514

22. 708
23. 326
24. 1,084
25. 4,205
26. 636
27. 1,864
28. 3,051
29. 7,576
30. 858
31. 5,625
32. 4,218
33. 13,084
34. 31,870
35. 113,880
36. 29,864
37. 556,470
38. 596,128
39. 743,445
40. 106,575

Practice Drills 3D

1. 10
2. 5
3. 4
4. 7
5. 5
6. 4 r 1
7. 12 r 1
8. 116 r 4
9. 418 r 8
10. 7 r 50
11. 131
12. 10 r 23
13. 16 r 24
14. 11 r 39
15. 1 r 5
16. 3 r 2
17. 5 r 3
18. 75 r 7
19. 26 r 1
20. 25
21. 1,508 r 3
22. 968 r 2
23. 1,417 r 5
24. 248 r 7
25. 1,374 r 1
26. 1,107 r 6
27. 896 r 4
28. 1,647 r 1
29. 653
30. 3,683 r 1
31. 239 r 2
32. 1,432
33. 484
34. 270 r 5

35. 923
36. 125
37. 541
38. 4,540
39. 17,820
40. 7,987 r 3

Practice Drills 3E

1. 26
2. 33
3. 49
4. 89
5. 23
6. 24
7. 79
8. 75
9. 36
10. 56
11. 14
12. 15
13. 96
14. 155
15. 120
16. 54
17. 16
18. 24
19. 88
20. 92
21. 45
22. 10
23. 20
24. 17.75
25. 11
26. 45
27. 10
28. 18
29. 24
30. 240
31. 104
32. 9
33. 8
34. 90
35. 133
36. 7
37. 32
38. 189
39. 99
40. 42

Chapter 3 Review Exercises

1. 35
2. 24
3. 33
4. 64
5. 5

161

6. 28
7. 48
8. 18
9. 0
10. 60
11. 108
12. 56
13. 154
14. 84
15. 940
16. 100,000
17. 2,664
18. 6,019
19. 17,860
20. 3,312
21. 24,321
22. 8,000
23. 1,920
24. 51,705
25. 162,916
26. 85,100
27. 230,770
28. 6,939,075
29. 13,738,618
30. 348,480
31. 4
32. 0
33. 5
34. 4
35. 11
36. 5
37. 211
38. 131
39. 16
40. 16
41. 4
42. 21
43. 84
44. 19
45. 38
46. 71
47. 0
48. 2
49. 17
50. 2

CHAPTER 4

Practice Drills 4A
1. proper
2. mixed
3. improper
4. mixed, improper
5. proper
6. proper

7. improper
8. improper
9. mixed
10. proper
11. proper
12. mixed
13. improper
14. improper
15. mixed
16. proper
17. improper
18. proper
19. mixed
20. proper
21. proper
22. improper
23. improper
24. mixed
25. proper
26. improper
27. mixed
28. proper
29. mixed
30. improper
31. proper
32. mixed
33. proper
34. proper
35. proper
36. improper
37. mixed
38. proper
39. proper
40. mixed, improper

Practice Drills 4A
1. proper
2. mixed
3. improper
4. improper
5. proper
6. proper
7. improper
8. improper
9. mixed
10. proper
11. proper
12. mixed
13. improper
14. improper
15. mixed
16. proper
17. improper
18. proper
19. mixed

162

20. proper
21. proper
22. improper
23. improper
24. mixed
25. proper
26. improper
27. mixed
28. proper
29. mixed
30. improper
31. proper
32. improper
33. proper
34. proper
35. proper
36. improper
37. mixed
38. proper
39. proper
40. mixed, improper

Practice Drills 4B

1. $1\dfrac{3}{4}$

2. $2\dfrac{2}{5}$

3. $\dfrac{12}{5}$

4. $1\dfrac{6}{12}$

5. $1\dfrac{4}{5}$

6. 1

7. $\dfrac{23}{4}$

8. $\dfrac{43}{12}$

9. $\dfrac{20}{7}$

10. $1\dfrac{1}{15}$

11. 4

12. $12\dfrac{2}{3}$

13. $\dfrac{31}{16}$

14. $1\dfrac{5}{20}$

15. $2\dfrac{22}{33}$

16. $\dfrac{28}{3}$

17. $\dfrac{42}{19}$

18. $18\dfrac{3}{4}$

19. $11\dfrac{1}{13}$

20. $\dfrac{103}{13}$

21. $\dfrac{28}{15}$

22. $1\dfrac{44}{55}$

23. $1\dfrac{1}{589}$

24. $\dfrac{64}{3}$

25. $\dfrac{56}{17}$

26. $3\dfrac{2}{5}$

27. $\dfrac{17}{5}$

28. $\dfrac{220}{213}$

29. $\dfrac{213}{7}$

30. $1\dfrac{6}{23}$

31. $\dfrac{2853}{273}$

32. $\dfrac{311}{100}$

33. $\dfrac{544}{111}$

34. $\dfrac{273}{52}$

35. $1\dfrac{10}{25}$

36. $2\dfrac{16}{24}$

37. $\dfrac{80}{24}$

38. $1\dfrac{16}{49}$

39. $10\dfrac{1}{20}$

40. $\dfrac{506}{5}$

Practice Drills 4C

1. $\dfrac{1}{2}$

2. $\dfrac{1}{2}$

3. $\dfrac{1}{4}$

4. $\dfrac{1}{5}$

5. $\dfrac{1}{9}$

6. $1\dfrac{1}{3}$

7. $1\dfrac{1}{15}$

8. $2\dfrac{1}{3}$

9. $\dfrac{4}{5}$

10. $\dfrac{3}{8}$

11. $\dfrac{7}{8}$

12. $3\dfrac{1}{6}$

13. $4\dfrac{5}{9}$

14. $3\dfrac{1}{4}$

15. $2\dfrac{4}{19}$

16. $\dfrac{1}{2}$

17. $18\dfrac{3}{4}$

18. $11\dfrac{3}{4}$

19. $4\dfrac{4}{11}$

20. $2\dfrac{1}{11}$

21. $\dfrac{5}{6}$

22. $\dfrac{1}{3}$

23. $\dfrac{6}{7}$

24. $2\dfrac{6}{11}$

25. $\dfrac{9}{14}$

26. $2\dfrac{6}{11}$

27. $\dfrac{9}{16}$

28. $2\dfrac{2}{3}$

29. $\dfrac{4}{9}$

30. $1\dfrac{24}{25}$

31. $8\dfrac{1}{3}$

32. $17\dfrac{3}{8}$

33. $17\dfrac{7}{16}$

34. $1\dfrac{1}{7}$

35. $5\dfrac{6}{7}$

36. $8\dfrac{2}{7}$

37. $14\dfrac{1}{2}$

38. $15\dfrac{1}{3}$

39. 25

40. $52\dfrac{1}{3}$

Practice Drills 4D

1. 1

2. $\dfrac{4}{5}$

3. $\dfrac{2}{3}$

4. 1

5. $1\dfrac{1}{8}$

6. $\dfrac{1}{15}$

7. $\dfrac{6}{17}$

8. $\dfrac{15}{94}$

9. $\dfrac{20}{21}$

10. $\dfrac{1}{7}$

11. $1\dfrac{7}{12}$

12. $\dfrac{2}{3}$

Module **Answer Key**

13. $5\frac{1}{3}$

14. $4\frac{2}{9}$

15. $2\frac{7}{20}$

16. $\frac{1}{22}$

17. $2\frac{11}{21}$

18. $2\frac{3}{104}$

19. $3\frac{23}{36}$

20. $5\frac{43}{45}$

21. $7\frac{5}{8}$

22. $1\frac{5}{9}$

23. $1\frac{5}{12}$

24. 1

25. $1\frac{2}{55}$

26. $5\frac{1}{6}$

27. $5\frac{1}{6}$

28. $2\frac{7}{15}$

29. $2\frac{19}{21}$

30. $3\frac{1}{30}$

31. $4\frac{17}{18}$

32. $3\frac{19}{30}$

33. $4\frac{7}{10}$

34. $3\frac{2}{35}$

35. $3\frac{29}{40}$

36. $8\frac{1}{15}$

37. $2\frac{43}{45}$

38. $5\frac{1}{8}$

39. $3\frac{11}{28}$

40. $3\frac{32}{35}$

Practice Drills 4E

1. $\frac{1}{5}$

2. $\frac{3}{16}$

3. $\frac{1}{5}$

4. $\frac{2}{9}$

5. $\frac{9}{32}$

6. $1\frac{1}{4}$

7. 2

8. $\frac{3}{4}$

9. $\frac{5}{6}$

10. $1\frac{23}{25}$

11. $3\frac{7}{16}$

12. $\frac{3}{4}$

13. $2\frac{8}{9}$

14. $10\frac{1}{2}$

15. $\frac{1}{105}$

16. $\frac{45}{154}$

17. $\frac{15}{28}$

18. $\frac{55}{256}$

19. $6\frac{177}{308}$

20. $38\frac{43}{64}$

21. $6\frac{6}{7}$

22. 4

165

23. $10\frac{1}{5}$

24. $21\frac{2}{3}$

25. 13

26. $2\frac{5}{14}$

27. $16\frac{1}{4}$

28. $1\frac{19}{20}$

29. $2\frac{19}{40}$

30. $1\frac{23}{40}$

31. $1\frac{23}{42}$

32. $10\frac{2}{3}$

33. $\frac{51}{80}$

34. $9\frac{5}{8}$

35. $1\frac{17}{18}$

36. $9\frac{1}{3}$

37. $1\frac{1}{45}$

38. $1\frac{7}{45}$

39. 8

40. $2\frac{8}{21}$

Practice Drills 4F

1. $\frac{4}{21}$

2. $1\frac{1}{3}$

3. $\frac{12}{25}$

4. $1\frac{4}{11}$

5. $3\frac{8}{9}$

6. $2\frac{7}{10}$

7. $\frac{4}{21}$

8. $2\frac{2}{5}$

9. $3\frac{17}{20}$

10. $6\frac{2}{3}$

11. $\frac{13}{25}$

12. $5\frac{13}{15}$

13. $3\frac{11}{15}$

14. $1\frac{19}{20}$

15. $\frac{22}{25}$

16. $4\frac{7}{12}$

17. $\frac{55}{72}$

18. $2\frac{5}{14}$

19. $3\frac{19}{27}$

20. $2\frac{3}{44}$

21. $2\frac{2}{3}$

22. $\frac{13}{15}$

23. $11\frac{1}{4}$

24. $8\frac{2}{5}$

25. $4\frac{3}{8}$

26. $6\frac{1}{9}$

27. $6\frac{2}{3}$

28. $5\frac{13}{15}$

29. $\frac{13}{25}$

30. $3\frac{3}{8}$

31. $3\frac{5}{9}$

32. $1\frac{7}{15}$

33. $3\frac{11}{15}$

34. $1\frac{19}{20}$

35. $\frac{22}{25}$

36. $4\frac{7}{12}$

37. $2\frac{5}{14}$

38. $3\frac{19}{27}$

39. $2\frac{3}{44}$

40. $\frac{55}{72}$

Chapter 4 Review Exercises

1. $1\frac{2}{5}$

2. $1\frac{1}{5}$

3. $1\frac{2}{3}$

4. $1\frac{4}{9}$

5. $\frac{1}{6}$

6. $\frac{2}{3}$

7. $\frac{19}{30}$

8. $\frac{3}{10}$

9. $1\frac{7}{10}$

10. $\frac{7}{8}$

11. $4\frac{5}{12}$

12. $\frac{7}{13}$

13. 18

14. $1\frac{3}{10}$

15. $\frac{1}{2}$

16. $1\frac{1}{25}$

17. $5\frac{2}{3}$

18. 2

19. $3\frac{38}{45}$

20. $18\frac{9}{10}$

21. $10\frac{3}{4}$

22. $\frac{19}{33}$

23. $\frac{5}{33}$

24. $12\frac{1}{5}$

25. $5\frac{5}{24}$

26. $6\frac{1}{12}$

27. $2\frac{5}{33}$

28. $\frac{5}{6}$

29. $3\frac{19}{20}$

30. $\frac{28}{45}$

31. $\frac{3}{35}$

32. $\frac{5}{18}$

33. $\frac{17}{49}$

34. $\frac{1}{25}$

35. $9\frac{3}{5}$

36. $\frac{19}{28}$

37. $\frac{12}{65}$

38. $2\frac{3}{4}$

39. $2\frac{2}{21}$

40. $\frac{7}{24}$

41. $\frac{1}{6}$

42. $3\frac{3}{20}$

43. $2\frac{1}{4}$

44. $1\frac{5}{11}$

45. $\frac{2}{15}$

46. 36

47. $1\frac{31}{74}$

48. $1\frac{47}{105}$

49. $\frac{75}{77}$

50. $1\frac{3}{32}$

CHAPTER 5

Practice Drills 5A

1. two and seven tenths
2. three and fifty-four hundredths
3. nine and seven hundred eighty-five thousandths
4. fifteen and seven tenths
5. fourteen and seventy-one hundredths
6. ninety-five and three hundred twelve thousandths
7. one hundred ten and twelve hundredths
8. forty-five and eight thousandths
9. three thousand three hundred eighty-nine dollars and fifty-seven cents
10. four million one hundred fifty thousand seventy dollars and ten cents
11. 12.4
12. 78.125
13. 103.002
14. 1,120.356
15. 17,894.12
16. 89.8952
17. $612.85
18. $2,400.40
19. $229,342.90.
20. 11,510.1265
21. forty-five and six tenths
22. three hundred twenty-seven and seven tenths
23. thirteen and seventy-six hundredths
24. four and fifty-six hundredths
25. eight tenths
26. twenty-three hundredths
27. three and forty-eight hundredths
28. twelve and seventy-nine hundredths
29. one hundred fifty-three thousandths
30. seventeen and five hundred ninety-one thousandths
31. 2.3
32. 6.4
33. 0.58
34. 0.701
35. 12.79
36. 44.46
37. 47.082
38. 282.505
39. 19.39
40. 3.1416

Practice Drills 5B

1. 0.01
2. 1.25
3. 0.8
4. 4.2
5. 3.4
6. 0.55
7. 0.36
8. 0.55
9. 1.75
10. 0.24
11. 2.6
12. 3.72
13. 4.06
14. 5.04
15. 1.4
16. 3.24
17. 5.12
18. 11.28
19. 5.875
20. 4.277
21. 3.2
22. 3.82
23. 0.58
24. 0.28
25. 0.636
26. 0.633
27. 0.636
28. 0.636
29. 0.85
30. 1.3
31. 0.76
32. 0.95
33. 0.6
34. 0.775
35. 1.22
36. 2.353
37. 0.555
38. 1.031
39. 1.587
40. 1.572

168

Practice Drills 5C

1. $\dfrac{1}{5}$

2. $\dfrac{3}{8}$

3. $\dfrac{4}{5}$

4. $1\dfrac{1}{4}$

5. $\dfrac{7}{100}$

6. $4\dfrac{1}{5}$

7. $\dfrac{8511}{10000}$

8. $2\dfrac{1}{4}$

9. $\dfrac{2}{5}$

10. $5\dfrac{3}{25}$

11. $\dfrac{3}{50}$

12. $\dfrac{3}{5}$

13. $4\dfrac{6}{25}$

14. $8\dfrac{3}{5}$

15. $7\dfrac{5}{8}$

16. $1\dfrac{7}{250}$

17. $9\dfrac{7}{8}$

18. $\dfrac{17}{20}$

19. $\dfrac{1}{8}$

20. $\dfrac{7}{8}$

21. $\dfrac{52}{125}$

22. $\dfrac{37}{100}$

23. $\dfrac{9}{10}$

24. $1\dfrac{4}{5}$

25. $3\dfrac{2}{5}$

26. $2\dfrac{63}{100}$

27. $4\dfrac{39}{100}$

28. $7\dfrac{7}{25}$

29. $\dfrac{3}{8}$

30. $6\dfrac{41}{100}$

31. $1\dfrac{372}{1000}$

32. $5\dfrac{391}{1000}$

33. $8\dfrac{29}{100}$

34. $11\dfrac{83}{100}$

35. $\dfrac{108}{125}$

36. $\dfrac{273}{500}$

37. $1\dfrac{29}{50}$

38. $6\dfrac{9}{20}$

39. $1\dfrac{43}{100}$

40. $1\dfrac{9}{100}$

Practice Drills 5D

1. 1.7
2. 12
3. 2.5
4. 64.09
5. 6.3
6. 156.9
7. 39.83
8. 46.63
9. 62.98
10. 36.29
11. 10.04
12. 329.3
13. 6.81
14. 4.33
15. 4.36
16. 17.74
17. 22.85
18. 33.65
19. 62.98
20. 226.82

169

21. 891.06
22. 349.01
23. 53.03
24. 793.18
25. 669.95
26. 742.4
27. 484.88
28. 924.44
29. 484.88
30. 219.75
31. 402.29
32. 18.24
33. 486.79
34. 12.16
35. 106.22
36. 41.08
37. 106.22
38. 85.95
39. 902.39
40. 703.23

Practice Drills 5E
1. 9.2
2. 6.44
3. 1.97
4. 12.54
5. 324
6. 524.52
7. 1.84
8. 40.87
9. 1.5
10. 83.98
11. 28.06
12. 1.61
13. 572.88
14. 756
15. 0.14
16. 30.45
17. 4.36
18. 10.89
19. 24,880.54
20. 8,093.21
21. 39.78
22. 10.65
23. -5.27
24. -3.57
25. -0.32
26. 26.79
27. 33.12
28. 68.76
29. -362.23
30. 109.08
31. 560.25
32. -30.62
33. 0.72

34. 71.71
35. 19.64
36. 10.91
37. 3.62
38. 2.81
39. 0.19
40. 0.07

Practice Drills 5F
1. 0.01
2. 0.8
3. 9.4
4. 3.2
5. 18
6. 4.4
7. 55
8. 6.39
9. 7.63
10. 9.1
11. 1.02
12. 23.19
13. 3,745
14. 2.49
15. 147.13
16. 1,207
17. 2,812
18. 62.5
19. 56.12
20. 0.03
21. 0.71
22. 0.17
23. 0.46
24. 1.27
25. 0.44
26. 4.96
27. 1.17
28. 0.48
29. 0.34
30. 0.07
31. 0.6
32. 2.04
33. 0.27
34. 0.77
35. 0.45
36. 0.38
37. 0.4
38. 0.11
39. 0.8
40. 0.75

Practice Drills 5G
1. 13
2. 72
3. 45
4. 20

170

5. 83
6. 13
7. 65
8. 20
9. 5
10. 17
11. 32.2
12. 66.2
13. 17.3
14. 53.9
15. 20.4
16. 0.6
17. 0.2
18. 0.1
19. 0.1
20. 0.1
21. 73.41
22. 19.13
23. 87.54
24. 52.36
25. 21.79
26. 49.79
27. 94.6
28. 7.35
29. 21.79
30. 53.11
31. 87.544
32. 52.359
33. 21.79
34. 49.789
35. 94.597
36. 7.345
37. 21.79
38. 53.111
39. 0.578
40. 0.051

Practice Drills 5H

1. 0.10
2. 0.55
3. 0.125
4. 0.28
5. 0.67
6. 0.2375
7. 0.0815
8. 1.33
9. 0.01025
10. 2.002
11. 20%
12. 35%
13. 15.5%
14. 12.5%
15. 15.75%
16. 9.5%
17. 0.575%

18. 75.5%
19. 150%
20. 250%
21. 0.2268
22. 0.5775
23. 0.0228
24. 0.1701
25. 0.01273
26. 0.496
27. 0.0038
28. 0.48165
29. 0.433
30. 0.03028
31. 3,218.9%
32. 6,621%
33. 1,725.6%
34. 5,393%
35. 2,036%
36. 57.75%
37. 20.35%
38. 5.06%
39. 10.23%
40. 9.66%

Chapter 5 Review Exercises

1. 22.12
2. 15.999
3. 0.987
4. 1.001111
5. 714.895401
6. $\dfrac{41}{50}$
7. $\dfrac{1}{4}$
8. $\dfrac{1231}{2000}$
9. $3\dfrac{1}{2}$
10. 1
11. 0.3
12. 0.625
13. 1.2
14. 2.6
15. 5.778
16. 19.48
17. 5.09
18. 13.704
19. 0.93
20. 13.222
21. 0.242
22. 72.82
23. 23.831
24. 173
25. 919.65

171

26. 6
27. 7.92
28. 11.27
29. 4.995
30. 12.07005
31. 38
32. 170.3
33. 18.5
34. 1.5
35. 28.1
36. 8.2
37. 5.9
38. 17.6
39. 0.9
40. 115.4
41. 1.01
42. 0.68
43. 0.01
44. 7
45. 15.62
46. 2.7
47. 5.75
48. 17.615
49. 25.112
50. 100.2507

CHAPTER 6

Practice Drills 6A

Convert the following to ratios.
1. 1:2
2. 4:5
3. 3:2
4. 19:10
5. 15:5
6. 3:4
7. 9:10
8. 5:1
9. 1:100
10. 1:1
11. 10:1
12. 1:10
13. 3:20
14. 1:2
15. 1:3
16. 1:7
17. 1:12
18. 3:5
19. 1:30
20. 1:5
21. 1:5
22. 17:20
23. 99:100

24. 11:10
25. 201:100
26. 10:1
27. 5:1
28. 1:15
29. 1:100
30. 1:6
31. 4:5
32. 1:2
33. 1:12
34. 1:5
35. 1:10
36. 11:25
37. 2:3
38. 1:3
39. 8:21
40. 36:63

Practice Drills 6B

Solve for x. Reduce to the lowest term.
1. 4
2. 6
3. 40
4. 12
5. 1
6. 5
7. 8
8. 40
9. 80
10. 14
11. 55
12. 3
13. 2
14. 12.5
15. 4.29
16. 7.64
17. 2.38
18. 15.86
19. 4.22
20. 167.75
21. 30
22. 13.33
23. 4.67
24. 1.71
25. 16
26. 1.5
27. 21
28. 3
29. 2
30. 8
31. 9
32. 34
33. 21
34. 9.88

35. 49
36. 25
37. 11.75
38. 17
39. 8
40. 20

Chapter 6 Review Exercises

 1. 2:3
 2. 3:10
 3. 3:2
 4. 1:10
 5. 10:3
 6. 3:4
 7. 1:25
 8. 13:20
 9. 23:20
10. 5:2
11. 1:4
12. 1:12
13. $\dfrac{5}{6}$
14. $\dfrac{1}{6}$
15. $\dfrac{2}{3}$
16. $2\dfrac{1}{3}$
17. $1\dfrac{4}{5}$
18. $\dfrac{1}{15}$
19. $3\dfrac{1}{6}$
20. 66.67%
21. 25%
22. 22.2%
23. 2000%
24. 750%
25. 2%
26. 250%
27. 25%
28. 250%
29. 0.3%
30. 3:4 = 9:12
31. 5:10 = 500:1000
32. 5:6 = 10:12
33. 3:8 = 15:40
34. 10:2 = 50:10
35. valid
36. not valid
37. not valid
38. not valid
39. not valid

40. 16
41. 8
42. 4
43. 1,000
44. 8
45. 2.4
46. 1.6
47. 6 cups
48. 28 pills
49. 12 loaves of bread
50. $45

CHAPTER 7

Practice Drills 7A

 1. 128 pt.
 2. 30 pt.
 3. 4 gal.
 4. 112 c
 5. 16 pt
 6. 4 qt
 7. 1 pt
 8. 16 qt
 9. 12 qt
10. 16 c
11. 41 lbs.
12. 432 oz.
13. 62 lbs.
14. 3 ft
15. 45 ft
16. 624 in
17. 6 yd
18. 12,992 yd
19. 1 mi
20. 2,376 ft
21. 566.4 oz
22. 8.75 gal
23. 1,233.6 oz
24. 997.92 oz
25. 54.25 lb
26. 0.38 mi
27. 0.26 mi
28. 1,214.4 yd
29. 3.34 mi
30. 2.03 mi
31. 1.05 mi
32. 0.10 mi
33. 3.58 mi
34. 42,240.16 ft
35. 74,448.28 yd
36. 0.13 lb
37. 32 oz
38. 9 yd
39. 0.3 mi
40. 100 qt

Chapter 7 Review Exercises

1. 14 lbs.
2. 52.5 oz.
3. 813 gr
4. $16\frac{1}{2}$ Tbs.
5. 215 gal.
6. 3 tsp.
7. 16 oz.
8. 128 Tbs.
9. 16 oz.
10. 19.2 oz.
11. 26 oz.
12. 24 Tb.
13. 16 cups
14. 600 drops
15. 48 tsps.
16. 32 Tbs.
17. 64 oz
18. 2,187.5 gr
19. 20.3 ℨ
20. 14,000 gr
21. 16 c
22. 0.5 gal
23. 24 qt
24. 16 qt
25. 1 qt
26. 12 qt
27. 31,680 ft
28. 8,800 yd
29. 624 in
30. 780 in
31. 20 ft
32. 37 ft
33. 36 ft
34. 135 ft
35. 11.7 yd
36. 34 yd
37. 72 yd
38. 3 yd
39. 780 in
40. 14 yds
41. 18 ft
42. 56 ft
43. 864 in
44. 27 lbs.
45. 608 oz
46. 40 lbs.
47. 832 oz
48. 3 lbs.
49. 6 lbs.
50. 816 oz.

CHAPTER 8

Practice Drills 8A

1. m
2. g
3. L
4. km
5. mg
6. cm
7. hg
8. mm
9. mcg or μg
10. dg
11. weight
12. volume
13. weight
14. volume
15. length
16. weight
17. volume
18. length
19. weight
20. length
21. liter
22. centimeter
23. kilometer
24. milligram
25. meter
26. kilogram
27. milliliter
28. microgram
29. meter
30. decigram
31. gram
32. centiliter
33. kiloliter
34. decigram
35. deciliter
36. dekagram
37. dekaliter
38. centigram
39. hectoliter
40. dekameter

Practice Drills 8B

1. 5 L
2. 15 km
3. 115 cm
4. 52 cg
5. 30 mL
6. 1,000 g
7. 0.001 mg
8. 50,000 mcg
9. 2.4 g

10. 49.9 kg
11. 5 kiloliters
12. 5 milliliters
13. 100 centimeters
14. 52 centigrams
15. 30 kilometers
16. 15 dm
17. 49.9 kl
18. 1,000 gr
19. 0.001 mg
20. 5 kg
21. 1.31 kiloliter
22. 2.64 hectometer
23. 100 milligrams
24. 3.53 hectoliter
25. 908 dekaliters
26. 0.27 millimeter
27. 125 centigrams
28. 1,546 centimeters
29. 10 dekagrams
30. 18 centiliters
31. 1.31 kL
32. 2.64 hm
33. 0.1 kg
34. 3.53 kL
35. 9,008 L
36. 0.27 cm
37. 1.25 g
38. equal
39. 100 hg
40. 0.0018 kL

Practice Drills 8C

1. 2,000 mL
2. 0.01 L
3. 1 kl
4. 0.046 L
5. 0.11 kg
6. 530 mm
7. 85 mg
8. 0.355 L
9. 1,600 mm
10. 0.109 kg
11. 9.5 dm
12. 2,000 g
13. 340 m
14. 10 L
15. 14,000 m
16. 0.250 km
17. 0.120 g
18. 0.455 L
19. 630 mm
20. 0.000043 kg
21. 1,310 m
22. 2,640 dm

23. 0.1 g
24. 0.353 kL
25. 9,080 L
26. 0.0000027 hm
27. 1.25 g
28. 0.01546 km
29. 100,000 mg
30. 180 mL
31. 0.0022 kg
32. 0.00003527 hL
33. 15,430 m
34. 0.0125 hg
35. 10,936 mg
36. 393.7 m
37. 0.0039 kg
38. 0.04 kg = _____ dg
    400 dg
39. 386,100 L
40. 155 kg = _____ dg
    0.000155 dg

Practice Drills 8D

1. 6.6 lb.
2. 10 kg
3. 6.8 kg
4. 4.5 kg
5. 19.8 lb.
6. 256 oz.
7. 154.3 lb.
8. 40 lb.
9. 30.5 cm
10. 152.4 cm
11. 274.3 cm
12. 274.3 cm
13. 91.4 cm
14. 13.1 ft
15. 1.8 m
16. 6.1 m
17. 2 in
18. 568.3 mL
19. 2 c
20. 16.1 oz.
21. 114.3 cm
22. 83 ft
23. 3.7 km
24. 35.6 cm
25. 56.7 kg
26. 75.7 L
27. 40.6 cm
28. 156.5 kg
29. 1.98 oz
30. 281.5 mi
31. 40.58 oz
32. 131.2 ft
33. 15.1 L

175

34. 354.9 mL
35. 110.2 lbs.
36. 7.5 in
37. 440.9 lbs.
38. 96.5 km
39. 12 oz
40. 453.6 g

Chapter 8 Review Exercises

1. 42.9 g
2. 625 km
3. 0.17 mg
4. Seven and five tenths centimeters
5. One-hundred two and fifteen hundredth milliliters
6. 42 L
7. 1,000 mm
8. 1 kg
9. 1 qt or equal
10. 1 yd or equal
11. 3.4 m
12. 1.95 km
13. 5 g
14. 3.6 m
15. 1.5 m
16. 2,800 mm
17. 1.3 km
18. 1.8 cm
19. 12 km
20. 0.0075 mcg
21. 0.000750 L
22. 500,000 mg
23. 3,750 mg
24. 0.0000055 mL
25. 0.12 cm
26. 0.6 L
27. 236.6 mL
28. 29.6 mL
29. 3 tsp.
30. 12.2 oz.
31. 5.4 kg
32. 20.3 oz.
33. 194 lb.
34. 119.1 lb.
35. 64 lb.
36. 92.6 lb.
37. 512 oz.
38. 1.8 oz.
39. 31.8 cm
40. 29.9 in
41. 7 yd
42. 6.1 m
43. 49 ft
44. 10.9 yd
45. 7.2 yd

46. 4.9 ft
47. 2 tablespoons
48. 6 teaspoons
49. 17.5 in.
50. 16.1 lbs.

CHAPTER 9

Practice Drills 9A

1. 32 °F
2. 212 °F
3. 14 °C
4. −9 °C
5. 1 °C
6. 29 °C
7. 58 °F
8. −4 °F
9. 49 °F
10. −38 °C
11. 13.3 °C
12. 150.8 °F
13. 92 °F
14. 31.1 °C
15. 39.2 °F
16. 35 °C
17. 188.6 °F
18. 38.1 °C?
19. 100 °C?
20. 0 °C
21. 77 °F
22. 113 °F
23. 32 °F
24. 68 °F
25. 194 °F
26. 104.5 °F
27. 149 °F
28. 38.9 °C
29. 2.8 °C
30. 93.3 ° C
31. 79.4 °C
32. 85 °C
33. 70 °C
34. 20 °C
35. 90 °C
36. 152.6 °F
37. 25.6 °C
38. 118.4 °F
39. 27 °C
40. 108.3 °F

Practice Drills 9B

1. 06:00
2. 02:45
3. 12:45

4. 11:30
5. 6:20 a.m.
6. 1:10 p.m.
7. 5:30 p.m.
8. 2:36 p.m.
9. 2:12 a.m.
10. 12:15
11. 11:45
12. 23:12
13. 8:36 p.m.
14. 13:25
15. 10:50 a.m.
16. 4:41 p.m.
17. 17:02
18. 01:56
19. 9:12 p.m.
20. 3:47 a.m.
21. 10:02
22. Morning: 10:02 a.m.
    Nighttime: 22:02
23. 7:15
24. Morning: 07:15
    Nighttime: 19:15
25. 2:40
26. Morning: 02:40
    Nighttime: 14:40
27. 23:15
28. 8:37
29. 21:25
30. 7:45
31. 5:53
32. 13:30
33. 10:15 a.m.
34. 7:38 a.m.
35. 11:05 a.m.
36. 8:45 p.m.
37. 1:00 p.m.
38. 3:37 a.m.
39. 10:30 p.m.
40. 6:36 a.m.

Practice Drills 9C

1. 120 minutes
2. 600 minutes
3. 6 hours
4. 9 hours
5. 3.5 hours
6. 615 minutes
7. 600 seconds
8. 960 seconds
9. 3 minutes
10. 5 minutes
11. 15 minutes
12. 48 hours
13. 4 days

14. 16 days
15. 312 hours
16. 1,800 seconds
17. 36 months
18. 156 weeks
19. 1,095 days
20. 94,610,000 seconds
21. 480 seconds
22. 120 hours
23. 240 hours
24. 540 minutes
25. 168 hours
26. 4 hours
27. 9 days
28. 6 minutes
29. 7 days
30. 5 minutes
31. 1 days
32. 8 hours
33. 71 hours
34. 14 days
35. 2 minutes
36. 360 minutes
37. 120 hours
38. 600 minutes
39. 825 minutes
40. 39 days

Chapter 9 Review Exercises

1. 25.7 °C.
2. 64.8 °F
3. 78.4 °F
4. 22.2 °C
5. 204.4 °C
6. 77 °F
7. 203 °F
8. 50 °C
9. 0 °C and 32 °F
10. 100 °C and 212 °F
11. 04:17
12. 16:50
13. 23:10
14. 00:59
15. 12:29 a.m.
16. 9:12 a.m.
17. 8:55 p.m.
18. 11:45 a.m.
19. 04:13
20. 7:05 p.m.
21. 2:00
22. 02:00
23. 14:00
24. 10:10
25. 10:10 (morning) and 22:10 (evening)
26. 20:10 and 8:10 p.m.

177

27.

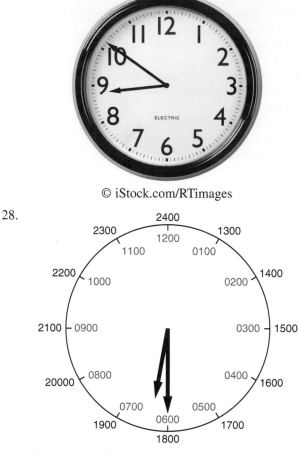

© iStock.com/RTimages

28.

2400
2300   1300
1200
1100   0100
2200   1400
1000   0200
2100 – 0900   0300 – 1500
0800   0400
20000   1600
0700   0500
1900   0600   1700
1800

Modified from Potter PA, Perry AG: *Fundamentals of nursing*, ed 10, St. Louis, 2021, Elsevier.

29. 240 minutes
30. 0.25 day
31. 18 hours
32. 64,800 seconds
33. 26 weeks
34. 182.5 days
35. 420 sec
36. 90 sec
37. 300 min
38. 10 hours
39. 5 h 5 min
40. 1 h 50 min
41. 11 h 40 min
42. 320 min
43. 130 min
44. 405 min
45. 42 days
46. 14 weeks
47. 7 weeks 1 day
48. 12 weeks 3 days
49. 30 weeks
50. 155 days

CHAPTER 10

Practice Drills 10A

1. Brand
2. Generic
3. Brand
4. Brand
5. Generic
6. Lipitor
7. 40 mg
8. 30 tablets
9. By mouth
10. 3 refills
11. 1
12. 5
13. 2
14. 6
15. 5
16. 5 mg
17. By mouth (oral)
18. Once daily
19. 30 tablets
20. 5 refills
21. omeprazole
22. 20 mg
23. By mouth (oral)
24. Once a day before breakfast
25. 90 capsules
26. 3 refills
27. hydrochlorothiazide
28. 12.5 mg
29. By mouth (oral)
30. Once a day
31. 30 capsules
32. 3 refills
33. Jane Q Public
34. John Smith, MD
35. Lipitor
36. 40 mg
37. By mouth (oral)
38. QD (once a day)
39. 90 tablets
40. 3 refills

Practice Drills 10B

1. John Smith
2. Dr. D. Haase
3. metformin HCL
4. 500 mg
5. By mouth (oral)
6. PO
7. Two times a day
8. BID
9. 120 tablets

10. 0 refills
11. nortriptyline HCL
12. Pamelor
13. 25 mg
14. capsule
15. by mouth (oral)
16. 30 capsules
17. PRN
18. QID or qid
19. 30 capsules for a 30-day month
20. 1 refill each month
21. clindamycin hydrochloride
22. Cleocin HCl
23. 75 mg
24. capsule
25. by mouth (oral)
26. 100 capsules
27. Q4H or q4h
28. 25 days
29. 1 refill
30. Lopressor HCT
31. 50 mg
32. 100 tablets
33. 50 days
34. 100 mg
35. ultram
36. 50 mg
37. 15 tablets
38. 4/2012
39. 5 days
40. 5 refills

Practice Drills 10C

1. 30 mg
2. 15 mg
3. 1 tablet
4. one tablet a day
5. 20 mg
6. 10 mg
7. 1 capsule
8. 2 capsules
9. 1,000 mg
10. 500 mg
11. 1 tablet
12. 2 tablets
13. 4 tablets
14. 2,000 mg
15. 2 tablets
16. 2,000 mg
17. 4 tablets
18. 0.8 mg
19. 2 tablets
20. sublingual (under the tongue) and PRN (as needed)
21. 3 tablets

22. 5 mL
23. 3 tablets
24. 2 tablets
25. 0.5 mL
26. 10 mL
27. 0.5 mL
28. 8 mL
29. 6 tablets
30. 4 tablets
31. 40 mL
32. 2.5 tablets
33. 0.5 tablet
34. 4 tablets
35. 24 mL
36. 1.5 tablets
37. 2 tablets
38. 4 tablets
39. 30 mL
40. 4 mg

Chapter 10 Review Exercises

1. by mouth
2. a patch on the skin
3. held inside the cheek
4. under the tongue
5. injection into the body with a needle or syringe
6. every day or once a day
7. three times a day
8. as needed
9. BID or bid
10. every 4 hours
11. lisinopril
12. 5 mg
13. tablet
14. by mouth (oral)
15. 30 tablets
16. 2 refills
17. QD
18. 5 mg
19. brand
20. 100 caplets
21. caplet
22. 500 mg
23. 8 caplets a day
24. 4,000 mg
25. 500 mg
26. 1 tablet
27. 8 caplets
28. brand
29. 25 mg
30. three times a day
31. 25 mg
32. 25 mg
33. 1 tablet

179

34. 3 tablets
35. 75 mg
36. 1,000 mg
37. 50 capsules
38. 12.5 mL
39. 125 mL
40. 5 mL
41. 150 mg
42. 7,200 mg
43. 1 tablet
44. 0.5 tablet
45. 2 tablets
46. 1 tablet
47. 2.5 mL
48. 187.5 mg
49. 1 tablet
50. 1.5 tablets

CHAPTER 11

Practice Drills 11A
1. oseltamivir phosphate
2. Tamiflu
3. By mouth (oral)
4. 25 mL
5. 12 mg/mL
6. 6.25 mL
7. 4 dosages
8. 2.5 mL
9. 10 dosages
10. 15 mg
11. 10 mL
12. twice a day
13. 300 mg
14. 0.25 mL
15. 4 dosages
16. 1.75 mL
17. 0.5 dosages
18. 20mL
19. 3,200 mg
20. 23 dosages
21. 10 mL
22. 0.5 mL
23. 0.4 mL
24. 2.5 mL
25. 0.6 mL
26. 0.75 mL
27. 0.25 mL
28. 1 mL
29. 10 mL
30. 10 mL
31. 20 mL
32. 3 mL
33. 10 mL
34. 0.5 mL

35. 8 mL
36. 40 mL
37. 24 mL
38. 5 mL
39. 6 mL
40. 1 mL

Practice Drills 11B
1. 420 mg
2. 16.8 mL
3. 52.3 kg
4. 627.6 mg
5. 12.6 mL
6. 320 mg
7. 12.5 mL
8. 6.8 kg
9. 68 mg
10. 2.1 mL
11. 272 mg (0.27 g)
12. 38.6 kg
13. 1,930 mg
14. 38.6 mL
15. 15.9 kg
16. 318 mg
17. 8 mL
18. 1,272 mg
19. 18,920 mg
20. 72 mg
21. 54.5 mg
22. 1,089 mg
23. 2 mg
24. 299 mg
25. 31.8 mg
26. 53.1 mg
27. 38.1 mg
28. 39.7 mg
29. 7.5 mg
30. 0.8 mg
31. 98 mg
32. 89.8 mg
33. 7.4 mg
34. 2.2 mg
35. 1.9 mg
36. 11.34 mg
37. 37.42 mg
38. 176 mg
39. 54.3 mg
40. 0.74 mcg

Practice Drills 11C
1. 2 mL
2. 4 mL
3. 4,800 units
4. 1,350 units
5. 1,363 units

6. 1,600 units
7. 1,288 units
8. 1.3 mL
9. 4,200 units
10. 4.2 mL
11. IV or SC
12. 5,000 USP units
13. 50,000 USP units
14. 6 mL
15. 1,200 units
16. 5,142 units
17. 51.4 mL
18. 1.5 mL
19. 5,273 units
20. 0.5 mL
21. 0.5 mL
22. 0.5 mL
23. 0.5 mL
24. 15 mL
25. 0.5 mL
26. 25 mL
27. 0.5 mL
28. 2.5 mL
29. 9.5 mL
30. 0.75 mL
31. 0.5 mL
32. 0.4 mL
33. 5.6 mL
34. 8 mL
35. 1.25 mL
36. 2.5 mL
37. 0.75 mL
38. 0.4 mL
39. 2.5 mL
40. 0.25 mL

Practice Drills 11D
1. Clark's rule
2. Young's rule
3. 36.7 mg
4. 84 mg
5. 235 mg
6. 95 mg
7. 66.7 mg
8. 20.8 mg
9. 128 mg
10. 72 mg
11. 86 mg
12. 73.5 mg
13. 11.4 mg
14. 17.9 mg
15. 160 mg
16. 16 mg
17. 60 mg
18. 4.8 mg

19. 200 mg
20. 206 mg
21. 37 mg
22. Clark's: 35.25 mg
23. Young's: 33.75 mg
24. Young's: 73.5 mg
25. Clark's: 66.7 mg
26. Young's: 17.9 mg
27. Clark's: 20.8 mg
28. Young's: 55.6 mg
29. Clark's: 86.66 mg
30. 16 mg
31. 0.4 mg
32. 184 mg
33. 17 mg
34. 160 mg
35. 11.4 mg
36. 128 mg
37. 96 mg
38. 5.9 mg
39. 909,091 units
40. 0.43 mg

Chapter 11 Review Exercises
1. 125.9 mg
2. 24.4 mL
3. 589.7 mg
4. 2.5 mL
5. 6.25 mL
6. 0.5 mL
7. 55.3 kg
8. 20 mL
9. 2,000 mg
10. 80 mg
11. 7.5 mg
12. 7.4 mg
13. 1.88 mg
14. 13,608 IU
15. 75,000 IU
16. 240 IU
17. 50 mcg
18. 1.5 mL
19. 150 mcg
20. 6 mL
21. 84 mg
22. 28 mg
23. 26 mg
24. 6.5 mg
25. 24 mg
26. 8mg
27. 5 mcg
28. 795 mg
29. 562.5 mg
30. 4.5 mg
31. 375 mg

181

32. Yes
33. 250 mg
34. 250 mg
35. Yes
36. 45 mg
37. 1.4 mL
38. 400 mg
39. 204 mg
40. No
41. 108.8 mg
42. Yes
43. 0.4 mg
44. 54.45 mg
45. 2.04 mg
46. Either by intravenous (IV) or subcutaneous (SC) injection
47. 5,000 units (IU)
48. 50,000 IU total in the vial
49. 9 mL of heparin
50. 4.8 mL

CHAPTER 12

Practice Drills 12A

1. 15
2. 8
3. 12
4. 395.4
5. 4
6. 10
7. 6
8. 54.6
9. 42.5
10. 31
11. 2.4
12. 68.3
13. 60%
14. 60
15. 7.5
16. 7
17. 10.1
18. 9
19. 6.8
20. 11
21. 7.1
22. 14
23. 13.1
24. 9
25. 9.7
26. 10
27. 9.8
28. 13
29. 14.8

30. 7
31. 24
32. 62.8
33. 22
34. 61 kg
35. 2.7
36. 171.6 pounds
37. 54 kg
38. 344
39. 64
40. 9

Practice Drills 12B

1. 5
2. 16
3. 27
4. 17
5. 156
6. 286
7. 91
8. 428
9. 8
10. 851
11. 4
12. 6
13. 2
14. 3
15. −2
16. 46
17. −10
18. −1
19. 1.5
20. 1.1
21. 4.2
22. 2.8
23. 2.5
24. 0.9
25. 2.9
26. 5.2
27. 4.2
28. 220
29. 0.5
30. 8
31. $81,330.33
32. 84.6
33. 23.8 miles
34. 4.5
35. 26
36. 7
37. 29
38. 75
39. 15
40. 50

Practice Drills 12C

1. 11
2. 6
3. 16
4. 12
5. 14
6. 5
7. 29
8. Mode: 70
   Range: 30
9. Mode: 8
   Range: 2
10. 9
11. 14
12. 16
13. 6.5
14. 14.5
15. 17.5
16. 10
17. 8
18. 52
19. 91
20. 21
21. 95
22. 16, 25
23. 20, 36
24. 51, 52, 60
25. Mode: 23
    Range: 8
26. Mode: 37
    Range: 63
27. Mode: 2
    Range: 9
28. Mode: 6
    Range: 11
29. Mode: 63
    Range: 8
30. Mode: 104
    Range: 13
31. Mode: 4
    Range: 9
32. Mode: 65
    Range: 54
33. Mode: 34
    Range: 16
34. Mode: 126
    Range: 21
35. Mode: 102
    Range: 20
36. Mode: 5.2
    Range: 1.8
37. Mode: 2.2
    Range: 1.5
38. Mode: 0.24
    Range: 0.64

39. Mode: 2.9, 5.8
    Range: 2.9
40. Mode: 125
    Range: 24

Chapter 12 Review Exercises

1. b. Median
2. a. Mean
3. a. Mean
4. c. Mode
5. d. Range
6. d. Range
7. 84.67
8. 85
9. 85
10. 15
11. 79.5
12. 89.2
13. 88
14. 79
15. 89.5
16. 29
17. 16
18. Mr. Barr's class
19. 13, 16
20. 14.6
21. 15
22. 3
23. 20
24. 41.4
25. 40
26. 60
27. 148.5 lbs.
28. 22
29. 3.7 lbs.
30. 81
31. 75
32. 17
33. 82
34. 83 or higher
35. 77
36. 99
37. 0
38. Sandra
39. Brian
40. Sandra
41. Mean: 57
    Median: 62
    Mode: none
    Range: 70
42. Mean: 51
    Median: 31
    Mode: 31
    Range: 67

183

43. Mean: 59
    Median: 60
    Mode: none
    Range: 85
44. Mean: 57
    Median: 59
    Mode: 59
    Range: 78
45. Mean: 44
    Median: 45
    Mode: none
    Range: 59
46. Mean: 54
    Median: 62
    Mode: none
    Range: 60

47. Mean: 55
    Median: 53
    Mode: none
    Range: 87
48. Mean: 62
    Median: 70
    Mode: 32, 94
    Range: 71
49. Mean: 55
    Median: 62
    Mode: 66
    Range: 75
50. Mean: 2,170.8
    Median: 1,211
    Mode: 1,211
    Range: 4,574

Answer Key

1. 858
2. $x = 326$
3. 1,474
4. 12.46
5. 560
6. 0.016
7. $\dfrac{1}{16} < \dfrac{1}{2} < \dfrac{10}{11}$
8. $45\dfrac{3}{5}$
9. 10
10. $2\dfrac{17}{35}$
11. $4\dfrac{2}{17}$
12. 2212
13. 0330
14. 12:45 AM
15. 37.9 °C
16. 71.6 °F
17. 0.005 g
18. 11,700 g
19. 198,000 mcg
20. 75,360 mcg
21. 2.69 kg
22. 99.8 °F
23. 99.8 °F
24. 2.3
25. 62 inches
26. 1.57 m
27. 56.7 kg
28. Pamelor
29. 25 mg
30. 30 capsules
31. 100 mg
32. Clindamycin
33. 75 mg
34. 100 capsules
35. 8 capsules
36. Subcutaneous (SC) injection
37. 50 mcg/mL
38. 6 mL
39. 12 mg/mL
40. 300 mg
41. 12.5 mL
42. 2.92 mL
43. 40 mg
44. 10 mL
45. 2,400 mg
46. 160 mg
47. 4 mL
48. 103.42 kg
49. 1,551.3 mg
50. 10.3 mL

185

Module **Answer Key**

Module   **Answer Key**

Module   **Answer Key**

Module **Answer Key**